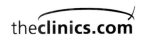

FOOT AND ANKLE CLINICS

The Diabetic Foot and Ankle

GUEST EDITOR
Brian G. Donley, MD

December 2006 • Volume 11 • Number 4

SAUNDERS

An Imprint of Elsevier, Inc.
PHILADELPHIA   LONDON   TORONTO   MONTREAL   SYDNEY   TOKYO

W.B. SAUNDERS COMPANY
A Division of Elsevier Inc.

1600 John F. Kennedy Blvd., Suite 1800, Philadelphia, PA 19103-2899

http://www.theclinics.com

FOOT AND ANKLE CLINICS   Volume 11, Number 4
December 2006   ISSN 1083-7515
Editor: Debora Dellapena   ISBN 1-4160-3863-9

Reprints. For copies of 100 or more of articles in this publication, please contact the Commercial Reprints Department, Elsevier Inc., 360 Park Avenue South, New York, New York 10010-1710. Tel.: (212) 633-3813; Fax: (212) 462-1935, e-mail: reprints@elsevier.com

The ideas and opinions expressed in *Foot and Ankle Clinics* do not necessarily reflect those of the Publisher. The Publisher does not assume any responsibility for any injury and/or damage to persons or property arising out of or related to any use of the material contained in this periodical. The reader is advised to check the appropriate medical literature and the product information currently provided by the manufacturer of each drug to be administered to verify the dosage, the method and duration of administration, or contraindications. It is the responsibility of the treating physician or other health care professional, relying on independent experience and knowledge of the patient, to determine drug dosages and the best treatment for the patient. Mention of any product in this issue should not be construed as endorsement by the contributors, editors, or the Publisher of the product or manufacturers' claims.

Foot and Ankle Clinics (ISSN 1083-7515) is published quarterly by Elsevier, Inc., 360 Park Avenue South, New York, NY 10010-1710. Months of issue are March, June, September, and December. Business and Editorial Offices: 1600 John F. Kennedy Blvd., Suite 1800, Philadelphia, PA 19103-2899. Customer Service Office: 6277 Sea Harbor Drive, Orlando, FL 32887-4800. Periodicals postage paid at New York, NY, and additional mailing offices. Subscription prices are $314.00 per year Institutional, $270.00 per year Institutional USA, $314.00 per year Institutional Canada, $253.00 per year Personal, $187.00 per year Personal USA, $209.00 per year Personal Canada, $121.00 per year Personal student, $94.00 per year Personal student USA, $121.00 per year Personal student Canada. To receive student/resident rate, orders must be accompanied by name of affiliated institution, date of term, and the *signature* of program/residency coordinator on institution letterhead. Orders will be billed at individual rate until proof of status is received. Foreign air speed delivery is included in all *Clinics* subscription prices. All prices are subject to change without notice. POSTMASTER: Send address changes to *Foot and Ankle Clinics*, Elsevier Periodicals Customer Service, 6277 Sea Harbor Drive, Orlando, FL 32887-4800. **Customer Service: 1-800-654-2452 (US). From outside of the US, call 1-407-345-1000.**

Printed in the United States of America.

CONSULTING EDITOR

MARK S. MYERSON, MD, President, American Orthopaedic Foot and Ankle Society; Director, The Institute for Foot and Ankle Reconstruction, Mercy Medical Center, Baltimore, Maryland

GUEST EDITOR

BRIAN G. DONLEY, MD, Vice Chair, Department of Orthopaedic Surgery, Cleveland Clinic Health Systems, Cleveland Clinic Foundation, Cleveland, Ohio

CONTRIBUTORS

SAMUEL B. ADAMS, Jr, MD, Resident, Division of Orthopaedic Surgery, Duke University Medical Center, Durham, North Carolina

LUCILLE B. ANDERSEN, MD, Assistant Professor, Department of Orthopaedics and Rehabilitation, Penn State Milton S. Hershey Medical Center, Hershey, Pennsylvania

VIKRANT AZAD, MD, Department of Orthopaedics, University of Medicine and Dentistry-New Jersey Medical School, Newark, New Jersey

GREGORY C. BERLET, MD, Assistant Clinical Professor, Orthopedic Foot and Ankle Center, The Ohio State University College of Medicine and Public Health, Columbus, Ohio

CHRISTOPHER BIBBO, DO, DPM, FACS, FACFS, Director, Foot and Ankle Service, Department of Orthopaedics, Marshfield Clinic, Marshfield; Clinical Instructor, Department of Orthopedics & Rehabilitation, University of Wisconsin Medical School, Madison, Wisconsin

PETER R. CAVANAGH, PhD, DSc, Virginia Lois Kennedy Chairman, Department of Biomedical Engineering, Lerner Research Institute; Staff, Department of Orthopaedic Surgery and the Orthopaedic Research Center; Academic Director, Diabetic Foot Care Program, Cleveland Clinic; Professor of Molecular Medicine, Cleveland Clinic Lerner College of Medicine of Case Western Reserve University, Cleveland, Ohio

JOHN DiPRETA, MD, Clinical Assistant Professor, Division of Orthopaedic Surgery, Department of Surgery, Albany Medical Center, Albany, New York

BRIAN G. DONLEY, MD, Vice Chair, Department of Orthopaedic Surgery, Cleveland Clinic Health Systems, Cleveland Clinic Foundation, Cleveland, Ohio

MARK E. EASLEY, MD, Assistant Professor, Division of Orthopaedic Surgery, Duke University Medical Center, Durham, North Carolina

JONATHAN B. FEIBEL, MD, Director of Foot and Ankle Surgery and Assistant Program Director, Mount Carmel Health Orthopaedic Surgery Residency, The Cardinal Orthopaedic Institute, Columbus, Ohio

ANKUR GANDHI, PhD, Department of Orthopaedics, University of Medicine and Dentistry-New Jersey Medical School, Newark, New Jersey

BYRON J. HOOGWERF, MD, FACP, FACE, Department of Endocrinology, Diabetes and Metabolism, Cleveland Clinic, Cleveland, Ohio

DENNIS J. JANISSE, CPed, Clinical Assistant Professor, Department of Physical Medicine and Rehabilitation, Medical College of Wisconsin, Milwaukee, Wisconsin

ERICK J. JANISSE, CPed, CO, National Pedorthic Services, Inc., Milwaukee, Wisconsin

THOMAS H. LEE, MD, Assistant Clinical Professor, Orthopedic Foot and Ankle Center, The Ohio State University College of Medicine and Public Health, Columbus, Ohio

SHELDON S. LIN, MD, Associate Professor, Department of Orthopaedics, University of Medicine and Dentistry-New Jersey Medical School, Newark, New Jersey

FRANK LIPORACE, MD, Assistant Professor, Department of Orthopaedics, University of Medicine and Dentistry-New Jersey Medical School, Newark, New Jersey

JAMES MATTIE, BS, Department of Orthopaedics, University of Medicine and Dentistry-New Jersey Medical School, Newark, New Jersey

TAMMY M. OWINGS, MS, Research Engineer, Department of Biomedical Engineering, Lerner Research Institute, Cleveland Clinic, Cleveland, Ohio

DIPAK V. PATEL, MD, MSc Orth, MS Orth, FCPS Orth, Chief, Department of Orthopaedic Surgery, Veterans Affairs New Jersey Health Care System, East Orange, New Jersey

TERRENCE M. PHILBIN, DO, Medical Director, Foot and Ankle Surgery, Grant Medical Center, Columbus; Assistant Clinical Professor, Orthopedic Foot and Ankle Center, The Ohio State University College of Medicine and Public Health, Columbus, Ohio

MICHAEL S. PINZUR, MD, Professor of Orthopaedic Surgery and Rehabilitation, Loyola University Medical Center, Maywood, Illinois

VICTOR R. PRISK, MD, Clinical Instructor, Department of Orthopaedic Surgery, University of Pittsburgh, Pittsburgh, Pennsylvania

VANI J. SABESAN, MD, Resident, Division of Orthopaedic Surgery, Duke University Medical Center, Durham, North Carolina

JAMES SFERRA, MD, Department of Orthopaedic Surgery, Cleveland Clinic, Cleveland, Ohio

CRAIG F. SHANK, MD, Department of Orthopaedic Surgery, Mount Carmel Medical Center, Columbus, Ohio

DANE K. WUKICH, MD, Chief, Division of Foot and Ankle Surgery, Department of Orthopaedic Surgery, University of Pittsburgh, Pittsburgh, Pennsylvania

CONTENTS

that foot ulcers precede most amputations. Certain ulcers will require surgical intervention to ensure healing, but all will leave the patient at high risk for recurrence. Here we review nonsurgical strategies for healing plantar ulcers and discuss approaches to secondary prevention. Effective offloading of the at-risk region of the foot is identified as critically important, and the value of appropriate therapeutic footwear is highlighted. A new approach to the design and fabrication of custom insoles is discussed.

When not treated properly, wounds of the foot and ankle can be devastating for both patient and physician. A multitude of wound healing agents are available, with some correlation to the type of wound or underlying disease, but for the most part the use of these agents is based on inherited common practice, personal preference, or marketing activities. This article reviews some of the most common products used as adjuncts to the healing process.

In this review, an in-depth anatomic and molecular pathogenesis of diabetic neuropathy is provided. Classifications and clinical manifestations of diabetic neuropathy are discussed. The current modalities of treatment and clinical research on this disorder are summarized.

Neuropathic ulceration and altered immune function place the diabetic patient at increased risk for polymicrobial osteomyelitis of the foot and ankle. The optimal method for evaluation and management of this difficult condition is controversial, and further studies are needed. Infected ulcers with exposed or palpable bone can be assumed to have underlying osteomyelitis. A multidisciplinary team approach is best, allowing optimal treatment of all associated conditions that commonly affect patients with diabetes mellitus. Empiric, usually broad-spectrum antibiotics and meticulous local wound care may achieve remission of mild-to-moderately severe infections and should be included in all treatment regimens. Severe infection, ischemia, or sepsis requires an aggressive surgical approach. Bone resection, correction of deformity, or amputation often are necessary and should be done with the goal of salvaging a functional foot.

(depth-inlay shoes and custom accommodative foot orthoses). It has been shown previously that as many as 60% of such patients can achieve this goal without surgical intervention. Many of the patients that require surgery have morbid obesity, an impaired immune system, chronic osteomyelitis with draining wounds, and localized osteopenia. Standard methods of internal fixation are applicable when these conditions are not present but are limited in high-risk patients because of the potential for mechanical failure or foreign body infection. Resection of bony infection, combined with correction of the deformity and application of a simply designed ring external fixator, may offer the orthopedic foot and ankle surgeon a stable construct with a low potential for mechanical failure, without the inherent risks of extensive dissection and the presence of a large foreign body in an otherwise compromised host.

Treatment of the diabetic patient with an ankle fracture presents a unique set of challenges to the surgeon. The care of these patients should follow a multidisciplinary approach. Meticulous preoperative planning, intraoperative technique, and postoperative care can decrease potential limb-threatening complications; however, complications will occur despite excellent care. Early recognition and treatment of perioperative complications is imperative. These patients require close attention for long periods, and the surgeon should plan on building a strong relationship with these patients.

FORTHCOMING ISSUES

RECENT ISSUES

THE CLINICS ARE NOW AVAILABLE ONLINE!

http://www.theclinics.com

ELSEVIER
SAUNDERS

Foot Ankle Clin N Am
11 (2006) xi–xii

FOOT AND
ANKLE CLINICS

Preface

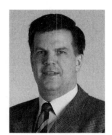

Brian G. Donley, MD
Guest Editor

Diabetes continues to be one of the leading causes of death and disability in the United States. Diabetes is associated with many long-term complications that affect almost every part of the body, not just the foot and ankle. Two hundred million people worldwide are affected by diabetes, and the World Health Organization expects this to increase to 366 million people by 2030. In 2002, diabetes cost the United States $132 billion. This is a disease that we see in our patient populations equally among men and women and occurs across all ethnic origins and races. Although the research continues on the management and treatment of the diabetic foot and ankle, the most important help we can provide our patients is the encouragement of healthy eating, physical activity, and monitoring blood sugars with proper treatment along with appropriate insulin management.

In addition to the significant difficulty patients have with their health, their disability, and the social impacts of their diabetes, these patients also contend with many economic hardships secondary to their diagnosis.

This issue of *Foot and Ankle Clinics* reminds us not only of the importance in treating our patients who have foot and ankle problems but also to have an understanding of the underlying effects of diabetes that causes the foot and ankle problems as well as the many associated problems.

Many of the foot and ankle problems we see in our clinics, whether diabetic or nondiabetic related, would oftentimes be treated best with prevention. This is certainly never truer than in the diabetic patient. We are provided in this issue with an excellent review of diabetes and its systemic effects, along with nonsurgical treatments that are helpful in preventing

doi:10.1016/j.fcl.2006.06.015

significant foot and ankle problems. In addition, this issue reviews many of the wound-healing agents that can be used to help our patients. Finally, for more significant problems, this issue discusses many advanced surgical techniques in the treatment of the diabetic foot and ankle.

I hope that this issue provides you, as it provided me, with a good understanding not only of the diabetic foot and ankle, but also of the overall systemic effects of diabetes and the importance of prevention.

Brian G. Donley, MD
Vice Chair
Department of Orthopaedic Surgery
Cleveland Clinic Health Systems
Cleveland Clinic Foundation
9500 Euclid Avenue
Cleveland, OH 44195, USA

E-mail address: donleyb@ccf.org

ELSEVIER
SAUNDERS

Foot Ankle Clin N Am
11 (2006) 703–715

FOOT AND
ANKLE CLINICS

Diabetes Mellitus—Overview

Byron J. Hoogwerf, MD[a],*, James Sferra, MD[b],
Brian G. Donley, MD[b]

[a]Department of Endocrinology, Diabetes and Metabolism, Cleveland Clinic,
9500 Euclid Avenue, Cleveland, OH 44195, USA
[b]Department of Orthopaedic Surgery, Cleveland Clinic, Cleveland Clinic,
9500 Euclid Avenue, Cleveland, OH 44195, USA

Diabetes mellitus (DM) is diagnosed on the basis of elevated blood glucose concentrations. Hyperglycemia associated with DM occurs as a result of insulin deficiency on an immunologic basis as with type 1 DM or as a result of impaired insulin action or insulin resistance as with type 2 DM. Secondary forms of diabetes may occur as a result of insulin deficiency owing to disorders such as pancreatitis/pancreatectomy or as a result of insulin resistance such as with Cushing syndrome or acromegaly. Complications may occur with any type of DM. DM is the leading cause of blindness, end-stage renal disease and nontraumatic amputations. Diabetes increases the risk for atherosclerotic vascular disease by two- to fivefold. Observational and clinical trial data show a clear relationship between the degree of hyperglycemia and the risk for diabetic retinopathy, diabetic nephropathy, and diabetic neuropathy. Intervention trials comparing two different levels of glycemic control show that for every 1% reduction in HgbA1c, there is approximately a 25% to 30% reduction in these complications of diabetes. Furthermore, data from the Diabetes Control and Complications Trial show that the effects of early intensive therapy are durable for periods of at least 8 years. Early detection for the complications permits early intervention. Other specific intervention strategies may also reduce the risk of progression of complications. These strategies include laser photocoagulation for diabetic retinopathy (proliferative retinopathy and clinically significant macular edema), blood pressure control, and modulation of the renin-angiotensin-aldosterone system (RAAS) for diabetic nephropathy and unloading devices for diabetic neuropathy. Lipid-lowering strategies,

* Corresponding author. Desk A-53, 9500 Euclid Avenue, Cleveland, OH 44195, USA.
   E-mail address: hoogweb@ccf.org (B.J. Hoogwerf).

blood pressure control, and aspirin therapy reduce the risks for atherosclerotic vascular disease.

Diagnosis

The diagnosis of DM is based on glucose concentrations [1]. The values as established by the American Diabetes Association were based on data associated with the risk of diabetic retinopathy—a complication essentially unique to DM. On that basis, the following criteria were established: (1) random glucose ≥ 200 mg/dL with symptoms, (2) fasting plasma glucose on two occasions ≥ 126 mg/dL, or (3) glucose levels after a glucose challenge of ≥ 200 mg/dL at 2 hours and at least one previous time point 30, 60, or 90 minutes after the challenge. It is well established that patients with fasting glucose values less than 126 mg/dL may have DM. Because abnormalities of glucose may be associated with coronary heart disease, risk and future risk of diabetes, criteria for impaired glucose tolerance, or "prediabetes" have also been established for fasting glucose concentrations between 100 and 125 mg/dL or 2-hour post glucose challenge values between 140 and 200 mg/dL. Additional criteria have been established for gestational diabetes, but these criteria will not be discussed here.

Types

DM may be broadly classified into type 1 DM, type 2 DM, gestational DM and secondary types of DM [1,2]. Type 1 DM occurs as a result of immunologically mediated damage to beta cells resulting in progressive loss of insulin production. Type 1 DM has a genetic basis with risk association for specific genes in the major histocompatibility complex on the short arm of chromosome 6.

Type 2 diabetes is associated with insulin resistance (related to central obesity) as well as progressive nonimmunologically mediated decline in insulin production. Although family studies, including high concordance of diabetes in monozygotic twins, suggest strong genetic predisposition, the genetic loci are not well characterized. There are environmental influences associated with type 2 DM including obesity (central), a "westernized" diet, sedentary life style, and probably sleep deprivation.

Secondary types of diabetes include those attributable to insulin deficiency associated with such disorders as chronic pancreatitis or surgical pancreatectomy and those attributable to increased insulin requirements owing to other hormonal disorders such as Cushing Syndrome, acromegaly, or pheochromocytoma.

Gestational diabetes is likely caused by glucose counter regulatory hormones that are associated with pregnancy and is associated with a risk of type 2 diabetes in the future.

Complications

The complications of DM include retinopathy, nephropathy, and neuropathy (both peripheral and autonomic). The risk for atherosclerotic vascular disease is increased in persons with DM. The risk for microvascular and neuropathic complications is related to both duration of diabetes and the severity of hyperglycemia. The increased risk for macrovascular disease antedates the actual onset of DM.

Diabetic retinopathy is a leading cause of blindness in the Western world and the leading cause of blindness in young people. Diabetic nephropathy is a leading cause of the need for renal replacement therapy (dialysis or transplantation). Diabetic neuropathy and lower extremity vascular disease combine to make diabetes the leading cause of nontraumatic lower extremity amputations. Finally, diabetes increases the risk for atherosclerotic vascular disease by two- to fivefold.

Strategies for detection, prevention, and management of complications all are important in dealing with patients who have DM. Key detection and treatment strategies for the complications of diabetes are discussed below.

Diabetic retinopathy

Detection

Diabetic retinopathy can be detected in the office with a handheld ophthalmoscope. This method of detection is limited by the area of the retina that can be observed and the fact that use of monocular devices seriously limit the ability to distinguish background retinopathy (vessel changes within the plane of the retina) from proliferative retinopathy (vessel changes that extend out of the plane of the retina into the vitreous). Similarly, macular edema may be missed by handheld ophthalmoscopy unless it is associated with retinal hard exudates—cholesterol/lipid deposits that occur in conjunction with extravasation of crystalloid and protein.

Adequate screening for diabetic retinopathy requires a dilated eye examination and should be performed by an experienced ophthalmoscopist—most commonly an ophthalmologist. Fundus photography can be used as a screening tool with properly obtained photographs, which are then read by an experienced reader. Stereo photography is required for best results. Technician training is required. This technique is unsatisfactory in patients with cataracts. Annual screening and regular follow-up as determined by the severity of retinopathy are the current standard of eye care in diabetes.

Prevention and treatment

Observational studies have found a relationship between the risk for retinopathy and integrated measures of glycemic control (eg, HgbA1c) [3]. Two large clinical trials have found that diabetic subjects assigned randomly to more intensive glucose control had a reduced risk for new onset retinopathy or progression of established retinopathy [4–7]. In the Diabetes Control and Complications Trial (DCCT), type 1 diabetic patients without diabetic retinopathy at baseline in the intensive control group (mean in-trial HgbA1c ~7.0%) had a 76% reduction in the risk for new-onset retinopathy compared with the conventional control group (mean in trial HgbA1c ~9%). Similarly, the progression of retinopathy was much less likely to occur in the intensive group (54% reduction) compared with the conventional group. Analyses of in-trial HgbA1c as a function of length of time in the study confirmed the concept that higher Hgb1c concentrations and disease duration were associated with greater risk of retinopathy (Fig. 1). The United Kingdom Prospective Diabetes Study (UKPDS) evaluated the effects of glycemic control in type 2 diabetic patients [5–7]. The intensive policy group had a mean in trial HgbA1c of approximately 7%, whereas the conventional policy group had a mean HgbA1c of just below 8%. The 0.9% delta HgbA1c in the UKPDS resulted in a 21% reduction in diabetic retinopathy.

For patients who have established diabetic retinopathy, the use of laser photocoagulation therapy has documented efficacy. The Diabetic Retinopathy Study evaluated the effect of scatter laser therapy in patients with proliferative diabetic retinopathy [8,9]. Eyes treated with argon or xenon laser had a reduced rate of progression of retinopathy and the associated visual loss. The Early Treatment Diabetic Retinopathy Study (ETDRS) evaluated patients at an earlier stage of their disease (advanced preproliferative diabetic retinopathy or background retinopathy with macular edema). Laser therapy was associated with a reduced risk of visual loss in patients with clinically significant macular edema [10].

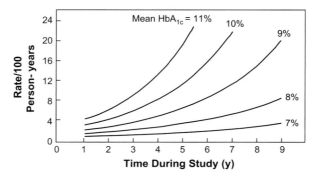

Fig. 1. Absolute risk of sustained retinopathy progression by HbA1c and years of follow-up in DCCT participants. (*Data from* Diabetes Control and Complications Trial Research Group. The relationship of glycemic exposure (HbA1c) to the risk of development and progression of retinopathy in the diabetes control and complications trial. Diabetes 1995;44:968–83.)

Future therapy for retinopathy

There is much interest in the mechanisms by which hyperglycemia may play a role in the development of diabetic retinopathy [11,12]. Among the considerations are interests in whether the accumulation of the sugar alcohol, sorbitol, might play a role. Sorbitol concentrations may be reduced not only by reducing systemic glucose concentrations, but also by interfering with the conversion of glucose to sorbitol, by blocking the enzyme aldose reductase. Studies using aldose reductase inhibitors have shown some suggestive favorable effects on diabetic retinopathy. More recently there have been investigations related to protein kinase C (PKC) inhibition. PKC is actually a family of enzymes found in many vascular tissues. Overactivation of PKC may occur in the face of increased glucose concentrations as well as increased diacyl glycerol concentrations. Increased PKC has been associated with micro vascular damage; the effect may be mediated through the production of vascular endothelium growth factor (VEGF)—a compound that stimulates the proliferation of new vessels. Studies of PKC inhibitors in diabetic animals have found a reduction in retinopathy. The studies in human subjects are not yet complete, but findings suggest improvement in vision even in the face of limited or modest effects on retinopathy. Most recently, intraocular injections of a VEGF inhibitor have shown favorable effects on proliferative diabetic retinopathy.

Diabetic nephropathy

Detection

Diabetic nephropathy is detected most commonly by using sensitive measures of urinary albumin excretion—commonly called microalbuminuria. The natural history of diabetic nephropathy is associated generally with a progression from microalbuminuria to a macroalbuminuria, which is then associated with progressive decline in renal function ultimately resulting in the need for renal replacement therapy. The American Diabetes Association recommends screening for microalbuminuria beginning 5 years after the onset of type 1 DM and at the time of diagnosis in type 2 DM [1]. This latter recommendation derives from the observation that type 2 diabetes may go unrecognized for many years before it is diagnosed.

Prevention and treatment

There are three major strategies to reduce the risk for onset and progression of diabetic nephropathy: glycemic control, blood pressure control, and modification of the RAAS with angiotensin-converting enzyme inhibitors and angiotensin receptor blockers. The DCCT analyzed the effects of glycemic control on the risk for new onset of microalbuminuria and progression from microalbuminuria to albuminuria. The group in which glucose levels were more intensively treated had a reduction in the risk for new-onset micro-albuminuria of 39% and progression to albuminuria of 54% [4]. In the UKPDS the 0.9% delta HgbA1c resulted in a 33% reduction in albumin excretion [5–7]. The early studies of the relationships of increasing blood pressure, increasing albumin excretion, and declining glomerular filtration rate (GFR) reported by Parving and others [13] showed the importance of blood pressure reduction in reducing the albumin excretion rates and attenuating the decline in GFR. Subsequently, modulating the RAAS with ACE-inhibitors and angiotensin receptor blockers (ARBs) has shown favorable effects on measures of diabetic nephropathy independent of blood pressure [14–20]. A recent systemic review of ACE-I and ARBs summarized the effects of these agents on mortality and renal outcomes from 43 published trials [21]. This review concluded that there were favorable effects from both classes of agents on measures of renal disease, but that ACE-I trials were more likely to show a reduction in mortality than ARB trials. There are tantalizing observational data that show relationships among dyslipidemia and the risk for diabetic nephropathy. In subjects from the ETDRS, elevated lipids at baseline were associated with a future risk for the need for renal replacement therapy [22].

Peripheral neuropathy

Detection

The onset of loss of sensation in the lower extremities is the most common symptom associated with peripheral neuropathy [23–25]. However, the onset often is insidious. Careful questioning of patients about loss of sensation or altered sensation to touch and temperature may provide clues to diabetic neuropathy. In addition, regular screening with a number of simple techniques has become the standard of care [26–28]. These techniques include testing for lower extremity reflexes, testing for vibration with a tuning fork (preferably 128 Hz), and some measure of touch usually with a pin or monofilament. Monofilament testing has become the gold standard. Patients need to be given instruction in the foot examination with special attention to development of callus formation and loss of skin integrity from foot ulcers, pressure-related blisters, or infections such as tinea pedis. Good patient care dictates a foot examination at the time of every routine visit to the primary care provider's office. Recognition of loss of sensation and early detection of foot lesions is necessary to help reduce the risk for neurotrophic foot ulcers or peripheral vascular disease—both of which contribute the risk for lower extremity amputations in diabetic patients.

Prevention strategies

As with the microvascular complications of diabetes, there is a clear relationship between glycemic control and measures of neuropathy. The DCCT intensively controlled subjects had a 60% reduction in neuropathy [4]. Similarly, the subjects in the UKPDS with the intensive policy had a 40% reduction in peripheral neuropathy as measured by a bioesthesiometer [5].

Patients who have evidence of peripheral neuropathy need to be instructed in a careful foot examination to detect callus formation, ulcer formation, or other threats to the integrity of the skin including blisters, cracks, or infections such as tinea pedis. Patients who have significant loss of sensation, especially with foot deformities and callus formation, need to be placed in footwear that will reduce the risk of further callus formation and the development of neurotrophic foot ulcers. Orthotic devices in footwear help reduce the risk of ulcer formation. Patients need to be instructed that even short periods out of the footwear increase the risk for ulcer formation in patients who have ulcers. Footwear that "unloads" the pressure areas is absolutely necessary for ulcers to heal. Patients are not often as adherent to consistent use of unloading footwear as would be ideal for ulcer healing. Therefore, the use of total contact casts has become one of the most effective ways to insure ulcer healing. Total contact cast application must be done by experienced technicians to avoid pressure ulcers in other areas of the foot as a result of the cast.

Painful neuropathy

One of the most distressing disorders associated with peripheral neuropathy is painful neuropathy. Often this is a self-limiting disorder. However, the associated pain may be quite severe. In addition to treatment with analgesics, other agents have been used in an effort to reduce pain [29]. These agents include systemic approaches (eg, amitryptilline, mexilitene gabapentin, topiramate, duloxetine) as well as topical preparations such as capsaicin. Each of these approaches is associated with approximately a 70% reduction in pain (compared with typical placebo responses of $\sim 30\%$). Because these agents work by different mechanisms, the clinical approach to treating painful neuropathy often includes sequential treatment with each agent in an effort to find what works best for an individual patient.

Diabetes and cardiovascular disease

Type 2 diabetes often is associated with insulin resistance, which, in turn, is associated with a number of cardiovascular risk factors. These include central obesity, hypertension, dyslipidemia (characterized by elevated triglycerides, low high-density lipoprotein [HDL] cholesterol and elevated small, dense low-density lipoprotein [LDL] cholesterol) a procoagulant milieu (increased platelet aggregation, elevated levels of plasminogen activator inhibitor I [PAI-1]) and inflammatory markers. When several features of the insulin resistance syndrome cluster together (obesity, hyperglycemia, hypertension, dyslipidemia), this has been described as "the metabolic syndrome."

Although there is not perfect concordance between the insulin resistance syndrome and the metabolic syndrome, for practical purposes, these terms often are used interchangeably. When components of the metabolic syndrome cluster together, there is a corresponding increase in the risk for coronary heart disease (CHD). The observational data from the Multiple Risk Factor Intervention Trial (MRFIT) screenees show that not only is diabetes associated with a two- to three-fold increased risk for CHD, but that risk factors such as dyslipidemia and hypertension confer additional risk as they do in patients without diabetes [30] (Fig. 2). Therefore, modulation of these risk factors should be associated with a reduction in cardiovascular disease risk. In fact, clinical trials of lipid-lowering therapy (especially LDL cholesterol lowering) and blood pressure control (especially with ACE inhibitors) have been associated with reduction in CHD risk [31–34]. The effects of glucose lowering on CHD risk are not yet well established in type 2 DM [5–7]. Aspirin use reduces the risk for atherosclerotic (composite of cardiovascular and cerebrovascular) disease risk based on data from the ETDRS [35]. (The primary purpose of this study was to determine whether aspirin [650 mg/d] versus placebo would reduce the risk for progression of retinopathy). These data are supported by the large observational study in those screened from the Bezafibrate Infarction Prevention Study. Aspirin showed a favorable effect in diabetic patients [36]. Further support for aspirin use in diabetic patients is reviewed in the technical review published by Colwell [37].

The first trial to test whether insulin sensitizer use in diabetic subjects (versus placebo) would reduce risks for vascular disease was the PROACTIVE trial [38]. In this study, pioglitazone was compared with placebo to determine effects on cardiovascular and peripheral vascular end points. There was no significant effect in the primary end point (cardiovascular

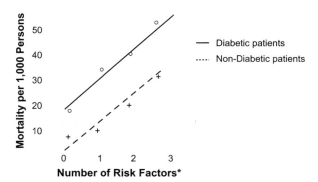

Fig. 2. Relationship of coronary disease mortality and number of risk factors in diabetic and nondiabetic patients. Solid lines represent diabetic patients; dashed line represents nondiabetic patients. *Risk factors analyzed were smoking, dyslipidemia, and hypertension. (*Adapted from* Diabetes Association. Role of cardiovascular risk factors in prevention and treatment of macrovascular disease in diabetes. Diabetes Care 1989;12:573–9.)

and peripheral vascular events), but there was a modest reduction in cardio-vascular events at 3 years (16% reduction, $P = .0247$).

Management of metabolic risk factors

Management of hyperglycemia, dyslipidemia, hypertension, and obesity begins with appropriate medical nutrition therapy [39,40] and a proper exercise regimen. In obese patients, even modest weight reduction usually has favorable effects on hyperglycemia, dyslipidemia, and hypertension. The American Diabetes Association nutrition guidelines recommendations to control saturated fat and salt intake are consistent with other published guidelines [41–44]. Carbohydrate counting with corresponding adjustment of premeal/prandial insulin is becoming a typical nutritional strategy for patients on insulin. Medication approaches to treatment of glucose, lipids, and blood pressure are discussed below.

Glucose-lowering agents

Glucose control in type 1 diabetes requires insulin therapy. Insulin regimen must include basal insulin; bolus insulin, which includes prandial insulin (to cover caloric intake—especially carbohydrate intake); and correction insulin (to correct hyperglycemia). Insulin analogs have become the standard approach. Combinations of long-acting insulin analogs (glargine, determir) and short-acting insulin analogs (lispro, aspart, glulisine) are used commonly now. Some patients may be treated with insulin pumps that deliver short-acting insulins on a continuous basis subcutaneously. Currently, insulin pumps do not have glucose sensors that communicate with the pump to alter insulin dosing ("closed loop" systems). Oral agents generally are not used in type 1 DM. Pramlintide, a synthetic injectable form of amylin, is a noninsulin glucose-lowering compound that is now available for use in type 1 DM. Clinical experience is limited, and nausea is a limiting side effect.

Glucose control in type 2 DM can be treated with oral glucose-lowering agents, insulin, or the new injectable synthetic incretins. Oral glucose-lowering agents fall into several general mechanistic classes including those that stimulate insulin secretion (sulfonylureas, repaglinide, neteglinide), suppress hepatic glucose production (metformin), improve peripheral insulin sensitivity (thiazolidenediones [TZDs]), or delay gastric emptying/glucose absorption (carbohydrase inhibitors). The typical range of efficacy results in HgbA1c changes in the range of 0.5% to 2.0% with most agents achieving ~1% change in type 2 DM. Agents that work by different mechanisms have additive effects, so combination therapy with two to four medications is common. Multiple combinations of medications are now available in a single pill (eg, sulfonylurea plus metformin or a TZD, metformin plus a TZD).

Side effects with sulfonylurea use include hypoglycemia whether used alone or in combination with other oral agents and occasional gastrointestinal upset. The risk for hypoglycemia is lower with the short-acting insulin secretagogues (repaglinide, neteglinide) than with sulfonylureas. Side effects with metformin include a metallic oral taste and diarrhea (~5% of patients). Metformin is contraindicated in patients with renal insufficiency. Side effects of the TZDs include weight gain and peripheral edema. TZDs currently are not recommended for patients with symptomatic heart failure. Side effects of carbohydrase inhibitors include gas and flatulence.

Incretin mimetics (exenatide, pramlintide)

Additional injectable glucose-lowering agents recently have become available for clinical use. There are gut peptides that stimulate insulin secretion and suppress glucagon production. Exenatide is an analog of glucagonlike peptide 1 (GLP-1)—a compound normally secreted by L cells in the small intestine. Exenatide stimulates glucose-dependent insulin secretion, suppresses meal related glucagon, delays gastric emptying, and suppresses appetite. Exenatide is approved for use in type 2 diabetes (absence of beta cell function in type 1 diabetes limits the insulin secretory effects). Exenatide use often is associated with moderate weight loss in obese patients. Nausea is the most common side effect. Native GLP-1 is degraded by an enzyme called DPP-IV, and oral DPP-IV inhibitors are under investigation.

Pramlintide is a synthetic analog of amylin. Amylin is secreted from the beta cells in conjunction with meal-stimulated insulin secretion. Pramlintide lowers glucose through noninsulin-mediated mechanisms and also suppresses glucagons and delays gastric emptying. It is approved for use in both types 1 and 2 DM and is given before each meal. Nausea is the most common side effect.

Lipid-lowering therapy

The primary approach to lipid lowering in patients with diabetes is to target LDL cholesterol reduction [41,42,44]. Statin therapy is the treatment of choice. Additional LDL cholesterol-lowering therapy including bile acid sequestrants or ezetimibe may be necessary in some patients. For patients with marked elevations of triglycerides, fibrates or niacin are commonly used. Combination statin plus fibrate or niacin is also commonly used. Side effects of statins are uncommon but do include muscle aches and liver enzyme elevations. The LDL-C target for patients with type 2 diabetes has been set at less than 100 mg/dL with a recommended alternate target in high-risk patients (eg, those with known CHD) at less than 70 mg/dL. If LDL cholesterol levels are at target, but triglycerides are still elevated, then a non-HDL cholesterol (total cholesterol minus HDL-C) is set at the LDL-C target plus 30 mg/dL.

Antihypertensive therapy

Combination therapy often is necessary to achieve adequate blood pressure control for patients with DM [1,43]. Current therapeutic targets set the goal blood pressure at 130/80 mm Hg. In patients who have microalbuminuria, blockade of the RAAS using ACE inhibitors or ARBs is the preferred approach. Otherwise, use of major classes of agents including diuretics, beta blockers, calcium channel blockers, alpha adrenergic blocking agents, centrally acting agents, and vasodilators all are considerations. In selected circumstances, possible adverse effects of the antihypertensive agent on glucose management or related disorders may need to be considered. Diuretics and beta blockers may worsen glycemic control. Beta blockers may impair the ability of diabetic patients at risk for hypoglycemia to detect the warning adrenergic symptoms associated with hypoglycemia. Often the benefits of blood pressure control with a selected agent (eg, beta blocker after a myocardial infarction) outweigh such adverse effects (eg, some impairment of hypoglycemia detection).

Aspirin

Aspirin therapy has been shown to reduce the risk for CHD and strokes [39]. There does not appear to be any significant adverse effects on diabetic retinopathy. Currently, the recommended doses for aspirin are similar to the recommendations for nondiabetic patients with daily doses of 81 to 325 mg daily.

Summary

DM increases the risk of multiple complications including retinopathy, nephropathy, neuropathy, and atherosclerotic disease. Management strategies include management of the associated metabolic risk factors such has hyperglycemia, dyslipidemia, and hypertension. Additional management strategies include laser therapy for retinopathy and appropriate footwear to reduce the risk of lower extremity amputations.

References

[1] American Diabetes Association. Standards of medical care in diabetes. Diabetes Care 2005; 28(Suppl.1):S4–36.

[2] American Diabetes Association. Diagnosis and classification of diabetes mellitus. Diabetes Care 2005;28(Suppl 1):S37–42.

[3] Klein R, Klein BEK, Moss SE, et al. The Wisconsin Epidemiological Study of Diabetic Retinopathy:XVII. The14-year incidence and progression of diabetic retinopathy and associated risk factors in type I diabetes. Ophthalmology 1998;105:1801–15.

[4] Diabetes Control and Complications Trial. The effect of intensive treatment of diabetes on the development and progression of long-term complications in insulin-dependent diabetes mellitus. N Engl J Med 1993;329:977–86.

[5] UK Prospective Diabetes Study (UKPDS) Group. Intensive blood-glucose control with sul-
     phonylureas or insulin compared with conventional treatment and risk of complications in
     patients with type 2 diabetes (UKPDS 33). Lancet 1998;352:837–53.
[6] UK Prospective Diabetes Study (UKPDS) Group. Effect of intensive blood-glucose control
     with metformin on complications in overweight patients with type 2 diabetes (UKPDS 34).
     Lancet 1998;352:854–65.
[7] Stratton IM, Adler AI, Neil AW, et al. on behalf of the UK Prospective Diabetes Study
     Group. Association of glycaemia with macrovascular and microvascular complications
     of type 2 diabetes (UKPDS 35): prospective observational study. BMJ 2000;321:405–12.
[8] The Diabetic Retinopathy Study Research Group. Preliminary report on effects of photoco-
     agulation therapy. Am J Ophthalmol 1976;81:383–96.
[9] The Diabetic Retinopathy Study Research Group. Photocoagulation treatment of prolifer-
     ative diabetic retinopathy: the second report of diabetic retinopathy findings. Ophthalmol-
     ogy 1978;85:82–106.
[10] Early Treatment Diabetic Retinopathy Study. Photocoagulation for diabetic macular
     edema. Early Treatment Diabetic Retinopathy Study report number 1. Early Treatment
     Diabetic Retinopathy Study research group. Arch Ophthalmol 1985;103:1796–806.
[11] Kaul CL, Ramarao P. The role of aldose reductase inhibitors and diabetic complications:
     recent trends. Methods Find Exp Clin Pharmacol 2001;23:465–75.
[12] Sjolie AL, Moller F. Medical management of diabetic retinopathy. Diabet Med 2004;21:
     666–72.
[13] Parving HH, Smidt EH, Methiesen ER, et al. Effective antihypertensive treatment postpones
     renal insufficiency in diabetic nephropathy. Am J Kidney Dis 1993;22:188–95.
[14] Lewis EJ, Hunsicker LG, Bain RP, et al, for the Collaborative Study Group. The effect of
     angiotensin-converting-enzyme inhibitor on diabetic nephropathy. N Engl J Med 1993;
     329:1456–62.
[15] Ravid M, Lang R, Rachmani R, et al. Long-term renoprotective effect of angiotensin-
     converting enzyme inhibition in non-insulin-dependent diabetes mellitus: a 7-year follow-up
     study. Arch Intern Med 1996;156:286–9.
[16] Kasiske BL, Kalil RS, Ma JZ, et al. Effect of antihypertensive therapy on the kidney in pa-
     tients with diabetes: a meta-regression analysis. Ann Intern Med 1993;118:129–38.
[17] Gerstein HC, Mann JFE, Pogue J, et al, on behalf of the HOPE Study Investigators. Preva-
     lence and determinants of microalbuminuria in high-risk diabetic and nondiabetic patients in
     the Heart Outcomes Prevention Evaluation Study. Diabetes Care 2000;23(Suppl 2):B35–9.
[18] Parving HH, Lehnert H, Brochner-Mortensen J, et al, for the Irbesartan in Patients with
     Type 2 Diabetes and Microalbuminuria Study Group. The effect of irbesartan on the develop-
     ment of diabetic nephropathy in patients with type 2 diabetes. N Engl J Med 2001;345:870–8.
[19] Brenner BM, Cooper ME, de Zeeuw D, et al, for the RENAAL Study Investigators. Effects
     of losartan on renal and cardiovascular outcomes in patients with type 2 diabetes and ne-
     phropathy. N Engl J Med 2001;345:861–9.
[20] Lewis EJ, Hunsicker LG, Clarke WR, et al, for the Collaborative Study Group. Renoprotec-
     tive effect of the angiotensin-receptor antagonist irbesartan in patients with nephropathy due
     to type 2 diabetes. N Engl J Med 2001;345:851–60.
[21] Strippoli GFM, Craig M, Deeks JJ, et al. Effects of angiotensin converting enzyme inhibitor
     and angiotensin II receptor antagonists on mortality and renal outcomes in diabetic ne-
     phropathy: systemic review. BMJ 2004;329:828–38.
[22] Cusick M, Chew E, Hoogwerf B, et al, and the Early Treatment Diabetic Retinopathy Study
     Research Group. Risk factors for the development of severe renal disease in the Early Treat-
     ment Diabetic Retinopathy Study: Early Treatment Diabetic Retinopathy Study (ETDRS)
     Report #26. Kidney Int 2004;66(3):1173–9.
[23] Partanen J, Niskanen L, Lehtinen J, et al. Natural history of peripheral neuropathy in pa-
     tients with noninsulin-dependent diabetes. N Engl J Med 1995;333:89–94.
[24] Vinik A. Diabetic neuropathy pathogenesis and therapy. Am J Med 1999;107(2B):17S–26S.

[25] Vinik AI, Park TS, Stansberry KB, et al. Diabetic neuropathies. Diabetologia 2000;43:957–73.
[26] Meijer JW, Smit AJ, Sonderen EV, et al. Symptom scoring systems to diagnose distal poly-neuropathy in diabetes: the Diabetic Neuropathy Symptom score. Diabet Med 2002;19: 962–5.
[27] Armstrong DG, Lavery LA, Veal SA, et al. Choosing a practical screening instrument to identify patients at risk for diabetic foot ulceration. Arch Intern Med 1998;158:289–92.
[28] Armstrong DG. The 10-g monofilament: the diagnostic divining rod for the diabetic foot? Diabetes Care 2000;23:887.
[29] Low P, Dotson R. Symptom treatment of painful neuropathy. JAMA 1998;280:1863–4.
[30] Stamler J, Vaccaro O, Neaton JD, et al. Diabetes, other risk factors, and 12-yr cardiovascu-lar mortality for men screened in the Multiple Risk Factor Intervention Trial. Diabetes Care 1993;16:434–44.
[31] Vijan S, Hayward RA. Pharmacologic Lipid-lowering therapy in type 2 diabetes mellitus: Background paper for the American College of Physicians. Ann Intern Med 2004;140: 644–9.
[32] Calhoun HM, Betteridge J, Durrington PM, et al, on behalf of the CARDS investigators. Primary prevention of cardiovascular disease with atorvastatin in type 2 diabetes in the Collaborative Atorvastatin Diabetes Study (CARDS): multicentre randomized placebo-controlled trial. Lancet 2004;364:685–96.
[33] The Heart Outcomes Prevention Evaluation Study Investigators. Effects of an angiotensin-converting-enzyme inhibitor, ramipril, on death from cardiovascular causes, myocardial in-farction, and stroke in high-risk patients. N Engl J Med 2000;342:145–53.
[34] The PEACE Trial Investigators. Angiotensin-converting-enzyme inhibition in stable coro-nary artery disease. N Engl J Med 2004;351:2058–68.
[35] Early Treatment Diabetic Retinopathy Study Group. Aspirin effects on mortality and mor-bidity in patients with diabetes mellitus—Early Treatment Diabetic Retinopathy Study Re-port 14. JAMA 1992;268:1292–300.
[36] Harpaz D, Gottlieb S, Graff E, et al. Effects of aspirin treatment on survival in non-insulin-dependent diabetic patients with coronary artery disease. Am J Med 1998;105:494–9.
[37] Colwell JA. Aspirin therapy in diabetes. Diabetes Care 1997;20:1767–71.
[38] Dormandy JA, Charbonnel B, Eckland DJ, et al. Secondary prevention of macrovascular events in patients with type 2 diabetes in the PROactive Study (PROspective pioglitAzone Clinical Trial In macroVascular Events): a randomised controlled trial. Lancet 2005;366: 1279–89.
[39] Franz MJ, Bantle JP, Beebe C, et al. Evidence-based nutrition principles and recommenda-tions for the treatment and prevention of diabetes and related complications. Diabetes Care 2002;25:148–98.
[40] American Diabetes Association. Nutrition principles and recommendations in diabetes. Diabetes Care 2004;27(Suppl 1):S36–46.
[41] Expert Panel on Detection. Evaluation and treatment of high blood cholesterol in adults. Ex-ecutive Summary of the Third Report of the National Cholesterol Education Program (NCEP) Expert Panel on Detection, Evaluation, and Treatment of High Blood Cholesterol in Adults (Adult Treatment Panel III). JAMA 2001;285:2486–97.
[42] Grundy SM, Cleeman JI, Merz NB et al, for the Coordinating Committee of the National Cholesterol Education Program. Implications of recent clinical trials for the National Cholesterol Education Program Adult Treatment Panel III Guidelines. Circulation 2004;110:227–39.
[43] Chobanian AV, Bakris GL, Black HR, , and the National High Blood Pressure Education Program Coordinating Committee. The Seventh Report of the Joint National Committee on Prevention, Detection, Evaluation, and Treatment of High Blood Pressure. The JNC 7 Report. JAMA 2003;289:2534–73.
[44] American Diabetes Association. Dyslipidemia management in adults with diabetes. Diabe-tes Care 2004;28(Suppl 1):S68–71.

FOOT AND
ANKLE CLINICS

ELSEVIER
SAUNDERS

Foot Ankle Clin N Am
11 (2006) 717–734

Pedorthic and Orthotic Management of the Diabetic Foot

Dennis J. Janisse, CPed[a,b,*], Erick J. Janisse, CPed, CO[b]

[a]*Department of Physical Medicine and Rehabilitation,
Medical College of Wisconsin, 7283 West Appleton Avenue, Milwaukee, WI 53216, USA*
[b]*National Pedorthic Services, Inc., 7283 West Appleton Avenue, Milwaukee, WI 53216, USA*

A successful diabetic foot care program focuses its efforts on prevention [1–3]. Two very important aspects of the preventive approach are education and the use of proper footwear [4]. Unfortunately, it is not uncommon for a patient to seek foot care advice only after he or she has already developed a problem, such as a diabetic ulcer. Often, these patients have never been tested for peripheral neuropathy or have not been tested recently, and many are altogether unaware of diabetic neuropathy and its associated risks [5]. It can be quite challenging to convince a person who has never had a foot ulcer or has not experienced foot discomfort to restrict their footwear choices to only those shoes that are considered by their health care provider to be appropriate. This task can be completed most efficiently when a diabetic foot care team, whose members support each other and collaborate in the best interest of the patient, undertakes it [6–9].

The physician and the patient are the people who form the foundation of the team, but there are many other ancillary but indispensable members of a successful diabetic foot care team. Other practitioners who work with physicians and their patients to prevent diabetic ulcers and subsequent amputations are certified diabetic educators, wound care nurses, physical therapists, certified pedorthists, and certified orthotists.

Total contact casting has achieved the status of a "gold standard treatment" for healing diabetic ulcers [10]. It should be stated for the purposes of this article that pedorthic and orthotic care are intended primarily as long-term management for maintaining healed ulcers and fractures and

---

* Corresponding author. National Pedorthic Services, Inc., 7283 West Appleton Avenue, Milwaukee, WI 53216.
E-mail address: janisse@execpc.com (D.J. Janisse).

for preventing future ulcers and fractures; in general this therapy is not considered the ideal treatment or healing option for open ulcers or active Charcot fractures [6].

The role of the certified pedorthist

Pedorthics is the art and science concerned with the design, manufacture, fit, and modification of shoes and foot orthoses to alleviate foot problems caused by disease, overuse, or injury [11]. Pedorthists fit and dispense foot orthoses, shoes, and shoe modifications according to a physician's prescription. A pedorthist is trained in foot anatomy, pathology, and the construction of shoes and foot orthotic devices. To achieve board certification, the pedorthist's qualifications are tested and accepted by the Board for Certification in Pedorthics (BCP). Board certified pedorthists are required to participate in a continuing education program under the auspices of BCP and are bound by a strict code of ethics [11].

The pedorthist plays a key role in the prevention of ulcers and amputations. The main area in which a pedorthist helps the patient is in providing appropriate and properly fitting shoes. This may include the construction of custom-made foot orthoses to fit inside the shoes or internal and external modifications to the shoes themselves. The pedorthist not only fits and dispenses these items but adjusts and maintains them as needed.

Another part of the pedorthist's role is patient education. The pedorthist is an invaluable resource for educating patients in shoe selection, including guidelines for proper fit, instructions for use, and appropriate materials and styles for an individual's feet. As a member of the diabetic foot care team, the pedorthist reinforces the information and instructions provided by the other team members.

The pedorthist also plays a part in the monitoring of a patient's progress and can be very helpful for follow-up between physician visits. He will also recommend follow-up with other team members as necessary.

The role of the certified orthotist

The word *orthosis* is derived from the Greek "ortho," which means straight, upright or correct. The term *orthosis* describes an externally applied device used to affect or change the structural or functional characteristics of the neuromusculoskeletal system. The words *brace* and *orthosis* often are used interchangeably, but *orthosis* is the preferred term. *Orthotics* then is the term used to describe the theory, practice, fabrication, and modification of orthoses, and a person proficient in this field is called an *orthotist* [12].

The orthotist is the member of the foot care team best qualified to provide ankle-foot orthoses. To become a certified orthotist, a candidate must show competency by passing a series of examinations administered by one of two certifying entities: the American Board for Certification in Orthotics and Prosthetics or the Board for Certification in Orthotics and Prosthetics. Like the certified pedorthist, board-certified orthotists must maintain a rigorous schedule of continuing education and adhere to their certifying organization's canons of ethical conduct.

An orthotist's role on the foot care team is much like that of a pedorthist's inasmuch as an orthotist is an excellent resource for patient education and for monitoring a patient's progress. Because the shoes and the selected bracing system must not only be compatible but complementary, the orthotist and the pedorthist work very closely with one another.

The roles of the pedorthist and the orthotist sometimes overlap, but more often each fills a void in the other's practice. While a pedorthist's scope of practice concentrates solely on the foot, an orthotist provides devices for the entire body. A pedorthist working in an accredited facility will maintain a significant inventory of therapeutic shoes and has an intimate knowledge of how each style fits; many orthotic facilities keep only a skeleton inventory of shoes on hand.

Shoes

Improper footwear has been shown to be a common culprit for causing diabetic ulcers [13]. Additionally, therapeutic footwear can play a significant role in lowering a patient's chances of foot ulcer development [7,14]. There are several objectives in providing footwear for patients with diabetes [15]. It is important to understand these objectives before discussing the different types of shoes or shoe fitting. They are:

- **To protect the foot**. An insensate foot needs to be protected from external sources of injury and the elements.
- **To relieve areas of excess pressure**. Repetition of high pressures during daily activities can lead to skin breakdown on the foot. These can be plantar pressures under prominent areas such as the metatarsal heads. They can also be areas of pressure over a bunion, a hammertoe, or a Haglund's deformity. Relieving these areas of pressure and redistributing the pressure more evenly can help reduce the incidence and recurrence of ulcerations.
- **To reduce shock**. A reduction in the overall amount of vertical pressure, or shock, is especially important for a foot with bony prominences or abnormal bone structure, such as a Charcot foot.
- **To reduce shear**. Shear is the fore and aft movement of the foot inside the shoe. The reduction of shear can help reduce callus buildup, blisters, and the heat caused by friction.
- **To accommodate deformities**. Deformities such as those resulting from Charcot arthropathy, plantar fat pad atrophy, and amputations need

to be accommodated. It is also important to consider forefoot deformities like bunions, bunionettes, hammertoes, and claw toes.

- **To stabilize and support deformities**. Many deformities need to be stabilized and supported to relive pain and prevent further destruction or
  progression of the deformity.
- **To accommodate foot orthoses and ankle-foot orthoses.** Foot orthoses
  and ankle-foot orthoses affect the way a shoe fits and must be taken
  into consideration. Not all shoes will accommodate such devices. If
  a metal bracing system is to be attached externally to a shoe, the shoe
  must be constructed properly to begin with.

Shoe types

Nearly every diabetic footwear prescription includes some sort of in-depth
shoes. Traditionally an in-depth shoe is an oxford-type shoe with an addi-
tional $\frac{1}{4}$ to $\frac{3}{8}$ inches of depth throughout the shoe [15,16]. These shoes offer
even more depth when the removable factory inlays are taken out. The addi-
tional volume afforded by an in-depth shoe makes it ideal for patients with
diabetes because it can easily accept a foot orthoses or ankle-foot orthosis
without affecting the fit of the shoe. The extra depth is also useful for accommodating deformities associated with the diabetic foot such as hammertoes
or bony prominences resulting from Charcot arthropathy. Off-the-shelf
shoes used for the diabetic foot are manufactured in multiple widths.

Other common features of in-depth shoes of special concern to those
treating the diabetic foot include shock-absorbing, lightweight soles and
strong, supportive counters. The uppers of in-depth shoes are made from
many different materials including cowhide and soft, supple deerskin.
Some have soft, heat-moldable linings that allow the leather to be heated
and stretched over a very precise area. There are also new synthetic upper
materials that breathe and mold like leather. A recent development in the
in-depth shoe arena is the introduction of stretchy elastic uppers.

There are a great many athletic shoes that are considered in-depth, have
removable insoles, are available in multiple widths, and are more cosmetically acceptable than the traditional oxford-type shoe.

When an off-the-shelf shoe is not appropriate because of extreme deformities or variance in size from left foot to right, it may be necessary to mod-
ify the shoe. If the shoe cannot be modified to fit, the last alternative is
a custom-made shoe. Custom shoes are fabricated by creating a positive
model—a "last"—from a mold of the patient's foot. The shoe then is constructed on or molded around this last. Because they are made directly from
molds of the feet, custom shoes offer the best possible accommodation and
protection but can be quite expensive compared with off-the-shelf shoes.
They also typically lack the cosmetic appeal of off-the-shelf shoes, and as
such noncompliance can become an issue.

Shoe selection

Shoe selection is based primarily on three things: the condition of the patient, the patient's foot shape and type, and the patient's daily activities. For a patient that has no history of ulcerations, shows no signs of peripheral neuropathy, and has a structurally normal foot, a properly fitting off-the-shelf shoe made of accommodating materials may be all that is necessary, whereas a patient with neuropathy and a history of ulcers, Charcot arthropathy, or amputations will require a much more complex footwear prescription. A patient with severe neuropathy needs a shoe made of a soft, moldable upper material and will probably require a shoe that will offer enough room for a custom foot orthosis.

The patient's body type is also a crucial factor to consider when selecting shoes. The construction of the shoe should correspond to the patient's body type. A large person needs a sturdy, well-constructed shoe that will not wear out quickly, whereas a small person could use a lighter weight shoe.

Feet come in all shapes and sizes; luckily so do shoes. The key component to both shoe selection and shoe fitting is choosing a shoe that fits the shape of the patient's foot. Not only must the shoe be of the correct shape to fit the patient's foot, but also it must be of the correct depth to properly accommodate additional devices such as foot orthoses and ankle-foot orthoses. The shoe needs to be appropriate for the type of foot as well as the shape. If the patient has a very flexible flat foot, then a stiff supportive shoe is in order. A rigid, bony foot requires a soft accommodating shoe with a shock-absorbing sole.

The shape of the shoe is dependent on the last over which it was made. Lasts are made in innumerable shapes, but the manufacturer determines the particular last used for any given shoe. Therefore, a size 7 shoe made by company X could fit dramatically differently than a size 7 shoe produced by company Y, as illustrated in Fig. 1 [16,17]. Lasts for therapeutic footwear are not only made in a variety of sizes but also widths and shapes. Some are made with a tapered toe, and others have rounded or squared-off toes. Other last shapes include inflare, outflare, and short- or long-toed lasts. Another useful option in therapeutic footwear is the combination last. A combination last is made with the heel significantly narrower than the forefoot [15]. This last allows plenty of room for the forefoot while maintaining a snug heel fit.

The depth of the shoe is important not only in the toe area but across the instep as well. The shoe should not put pressure across the dorsum of the foot. Additionally, shoes with laces or hook-and-loop closure systems generally fit better than slip-on shoes. Persons with neuropathy should avoid slip-on shoes because they are, by design, too short and too tight.

The patient's occupation, level of ambulation, and other environmental factors come into play when choosing a shoe style. Certain jobs require the employee to wear steel-toed safety shoes or boots, whereas others demand formal dress shoes.

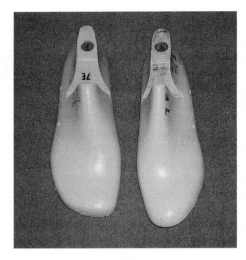

Fig. 1. Both of the lasts shown here are size 7E, made for the same shoe manufacturer, but a shoe made on each of these lasts will clearly not fit the same foot.

Shoe fitting

Once a properly shaped shoe has been selected, the next step is determining the appropriate size. There are several devices for assessing shoe size, but the Brannock device is the most complete (Fig. 2). The Brannock measures overall foot length, arch length (heel-to-ball) and width [17]. The proper shoe size is the one that ultimately insures that the first metatarsophalangeal

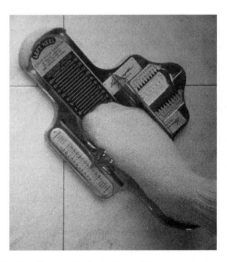

Fig. 2. The Brannock device is used to measure foot size.

joint is seated comfortably in the widest part of the shoe. This is why arch length is such a valuable measure.

The foot should be measured both weight bearing and non–weight bearing to evaluate how much the foot shape and size changes. Also, both feet should be measured because most people have one foot longer than the other [18]. If this difference is significant, a pair of mismated shoes may be in order.

Measuring the foot by any means determines just that—the size of the foot. This measurement does not necessarily correspond directly to the shoe size. It is up to the pedorthist to know his or her inventory and have an intimate knowledge of how each different shoe fits, how each corresponds to the foot measurement, and each shoe's fitting intricacies and idiosyncrasies.

A properly fitted shoe will have $\frac{3}{8}$ to $\frac{1}{2}$ inch between the end of the longest toe and the front of the shoe [16,17,19]. The shoe should also allow for a small amount of movement of the heel because the foot stretches and the calcaneous shifts during gait. Also, the upper material should not be stretched taut across the ball of the foot; there should be appreciable slack in the material.

Properly fitting shoes are essential to preventing foot problems, yet a large percentage of the population wears ill-fitting shoes [20]. Education on and understanding of proper shoe fit is crucial.

Foot orthoses will be discussed in the following section, but for all of the attention garnered by orthoses, it is imperative to remember that the orthosis is only as good as the shoe in which it is worn [21].

Foot orthoses

Foot orthoses are also an important component in preventing foot ulcerations [22]. Foot orthoses are available as custom-made devices, made directly from a mold or model of the patient's foot, or they can be prefabricated, off-the-shelf devices. Both can be made from a variety of materials differing in density, cushioning, shock absorption, support, and control. By using a prefabricated device, one significantly reduces the cost and time investment of both practitioner and patient but sacrifices the intimate fit, longevity, and adjustability of a custom device. For this reason, a custom device is necessary for any patient who has any of the following: a significant degree of deformity, a loss of protective sensation, or a history of ulcers or Charcot arthropathy. A custom foot orthosis can achieve total contact with the plantar surface of the patient's foot, therefore, using the same total contact concept as the total concept cast [23].

Although there are four main types of custom foot orthoses, it is imperative to remember that not all are indicated for use in patients with diabetic neuropathy. The four types of orthoses are accommodative, semirigid, rigid, and the partial foot prosthesis. All except the partial foot prosthesis are available in off-the-shelf versions as well.

To provide the patient with the best possible orthosis, the practitioner needs to understand lower limb biomechanics and be able to identify areas of high pressure; they also need to use the proper molding technique and be able to select the best material given the desired function of the orthosis [24].

When using a foot orthoses for treatment of the diabetic foot, one of the primary functions of the orthosis is to cushion and protect the foot. Additionally, the following component objectives of a foot orthosis should be to [15,24]:

- Provide shock absorption and shock attenuation
- Relieve areas of high plantar pressure by evenly redistributing weight-bearing pressures over the entire plantar surface
- Support, splint, and protect healed fractures sites by using the total contact concept
- Reduce shear through the use of the total contact concept
- Control, stabilize, support, or correct flexible deformities through the use of combinations of soft and semirigid materials
- Limit the motion of joints through the use of combinations of soft and semirigid materials
- Accommodate fixed deformities by using soft, moldable materials

Accommodative foot orthoses

An accommodative foot orthosis is designed primarily to cushion and protect the foot. It offers good shock absorption and ample padding. It can be designed to offload prominent areas. An accommodative orthosis typically is not one that will perform at a high level for a long period. Softer, less dense materials tend to wear out quickly, so this type of orthosis requires vigilant follow-up and needs to be repaired or replaced on a regular basis. This type of orthosis is good for someone who has very little or no deformity; is not a large, active person; and who needs only preventive padding in their shoes.

Depending on the materials used, accommodative orthoses can be molded directly to the patient's foot using either external heat and pressure or the patient's own body heat and weight to mold them. Accommodative orthoses also can be fabricated over a positive model of the patient's foot. This model could be a plaster model made from a negative mold of the person's foot or a computer-generated model based on a three-dimensional scan. There are three principal ways to create a positive model of the patient's foot:

- Foam box—A box of crushable foam is used to obtain an impression of the patient's foot. The void created in the foam is then filled with plaster to make a replica of the patient's foot.

- Plaster cast—A traditional plaster cast is applied to the foot while the foot is held in the desired position. The resulting plaster shell is then filled with plaster to make a replica of the patient's foot.
- CAD-CAM—The foot is scanned by a computerized system to create a virtual model of the patient's foot. This information is then relayed to a milling machine that mills out an orthosis to mirror the bottom of the patient's foot. Turnaround time for CAD-CAM orthoses can be as fast as same-day. One major criticism of the CAD-CAM is the limited selection of orthosis materials available for milling [21].

Accommodative foot orthoses are made of soft, moldable materials. The following is a list of materials commonly used to fabricate accommodative orthoses:

- Soft cross-linked polyethylene foams. These foams are heat-moldable and very soft. However, when used alone, they compress very quickly to a point at which they can no longer compress—they are bottomed out—and are then useless from a functional standpoint [24].
- Open-cell polyurethane foams. These materials are very good for reducing shear and absorbing shock. They do not bottom out quickly, thus adding longevity to an orthotic device. The drawback to polyurethane foams is that they are not heat moldable. If they are to be used in an orthosis they must be backed with or sandwiched between heat-moldable materials.
- Sponge rubber. Sponge rubber is available in varying densities and does not bottom out rapidly. Like the polyurethane foams, it is not heat moldable.
- Closed-cell expanded rubber. This material is very useful because it can maintain up to 90% of its thickness under heavy loads. The negatives are that it cannot be heat molded and it may be allergenic.

In general terms, the moldable materials possess better pressure distribution properties than the nonmoldable materials, but they are not as durable and bottom out more rapidly [25].

Semirigid foot orthoses

Semirigid foot orthoses combine the cushion and protection of the accommodative orthoses with the support, control, and weight redistribution of the rigid orthoses. Semirigid orthoses offer much greater longevity than the accommodative orthoses.

A semirigid orthoses for a patient with diabetes typically consists of a soft, cushioned protective top layer with a firmer, more supportive base material. The rigid orthosis supports the foot by using a thin layer of firm, inflexible material, and the semi-rigid device relies on a thicker layer of a semiflexible material that offers support as well as shock absorption and cushion.

The molding techniques described above all can be used to create semirigid orthoses, with the foam box and the CAD-CAM systems being more commonly used.

The concept behind the semirigid device is that to alleviate areas of high pressure and prevent skin breakdown, it is necessary to redistribute and equilibrate plantar pressures. The soft materials in an accommodative orthoses accomplish this goal for only a short period because the soft materials compress rapidly under areas of high pressure, thereby quickly returning those areas to their previous state of elevated pressures. By using a firmer material to support the arch and cradle the heel, the soft materials in the top cover of a semirigid device do not compress as rapidly, and the plantar pressures are distributed more evenly [24]. In an insensate foot, the areas of highest pressure are typically under the heel and the ball of the foot [26]. With a weight-redistributing, total contact, semirigid foot orthosis, the entire plantar surface of the foot participates in the weight-bearing process (Fig. 3).

A semirigid orthosis is also an invaluable tool for offloading plantar prominences like dropped metatarsal heads or bony prominences that are the result of Charcot arthropathy.

The top layer or layers of a diabetic semirigid orthosis generally consist of thin layers of accommodative materials. Semirigid orthoses typically are made of combinations of two, three, four or more different materials. The following is a list of some of the commonly used semirigid foot orthoses materials used to make the solid base of the device:

- Firm cross-linked polyethylene foams. These closed-cell materials are heat moldable and conform quickly to the shape of the foot. They have very good shock absorbing qualities and are available in a variety of densities.
- Ethylene vinyl acetates. These materials are also heat moldable. Because their cells are smaller than the polyethylene foams, they last longer and hold up better under weight. They are also good shock absorbers.

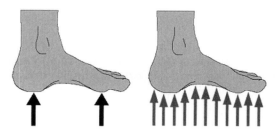

Fig. 3. In normal weight bearing most of the pressure is under the heel and ball of the foot, as illustrated by the drawing on the left. With a foot orthotic, the pressure is distributed more evenly as shown in the drawing on the right.

- Cork composites. This class of materials contains many different cork-based composites made up of cork and any or all of the following: plastic, rubber, fiberglass, and ethylene vinyl acetate. Cork composites can be very lightweight. They typically are good shock absorbers and do not compress quickly. They offer strong support without sacrificing cushion.

Semirigid orthoses are almost infinitely adjustable and can be modified to accommodate changes in the foot. These devices require consistent follow-up and will need to be replaced annually.

A study by Brodsky and colleagues [25] of five commonly used foot orthosis materials found that the soft polyethylene foams had better pressure-distribution characteristics when first applied, but that exposure to repeated pressures caused them to bottom out more rapidly than some of the more durable polymers. Other studies give credence to this concept and also show that loss of thickness of the molded polyurethane foam is inversely related to its density [27,28]. These findings suggest that to achieve the total contact objective as well as provide adequate shock absorption and support, a foot orthosis for use in treating the diabetic foot should be comprised of a combination of materials. A triple-layer molded orthosis has been suggested to provide the necessary combination of support and accommodation [24,29]. The three layers would then be:

1. Soft, moldable polyethylene foam next to the foot.
2. A middle layer consisting of a urethane polymer that resists bottoming out and offers good shock absorption.
3. A firm, molded cork or dense ethylene vinyl acetate base for support and control.

Orthoses made of material with excellent shock absorbing qualities, such as a viscoelastic polymer, have been shown to reduce significantly the abnormally high plantar pressures of a diabetic foot [30].

Rigid foot orthoses

Rigid orthoses generally are contraindicated for persons with diabetes, especially if there is evidence of neuropathy or a history of ulcerations. They can be extremely difficult to fit [31]. Rigid orthoses are not forgiving and do not mold or conform to prominences on the plantar surface of the foot; therefore, they may cause injury [21].

Rigid orthoses often are made of thermoplastics, acrylics, or carbon fiber composites. They are not easily adjustable. Rigid orthoses are durable and offer excellent support and control but provide very little in the way of cushion, shock absorption, and protection [29]. In some cases, they can be more of a hazard than an aid.

Partial foot prosthesis

A seemingly unavoidable aspect of caring for persons with diabetes is the need to address the partially amputated foot. This is accomplished through the use of a semirigid device with an accommodative top cover and a soft buffer material between the orthosis and the foot remnant. The device is molded around a model of the foot and the void at which the amputated portion was is filled in using a firm material [32].

Off-the-shelf orthoses

Off-the-shelf orthoses can be used as a suitable preventive measure when the patient has no deformity, neuropathy, or ulcers [31]. They are a less expensive alternative to custom devices, but if a patient has a history of ulcerations or sensory limitations, custom orthoses are necessary.

Bracing options

The main functions of bracing in the diabetic foot are to correct deformity, reduce or eliminate motion, decrease stresses to the foot and ankle, and transfer forces [31].

The three main types of braces used in the care of the diabetic foot are:

1. Molded plastic ankle foot orthosis (AFO)
2. Metal hybrid attached to shoe
3. Charcot restraint orthotic walker (CROW)

A molded AFO can be used to control medial-lateral motion but more importantly to control dorsiflexion and plantarflexion [33].A molded AFO is particularly useful because it fits inside a shoe. It will have its own molded footbed, so there is no need for an additional foot orthoses. The molded AFO is a valuable tool for protecting a Charcot foot after the arthropathic process has subsided [34]. It also is useful for reducing stress on the midfoot and hindfoot joints after an ankle fusion. The molded AFO often is the most cosmetically acceptable bracing option. The molded AFO is much lighter than the metal bracing systems, but can create more complex shoe fitting issues. Thermoplastics such as polypropylene or copolymer polypropylene are used commonly to fabricate molded AFOs.

A metal hybrid has the advantage of variable joints at the ankle, thereby allowing for free motion to a certain set degree while limiting harmful motion. For example, if the objective is to decrease bending forces across the midfoot, the practitioner would set the hinge to allow full plantarflexion but stop dorsiflexion at 90°. This joint setting, when used with a strong, wide stirrup and an extended steel shank and rocker sole in the shoe can reduce the bending forces seen at the midfoot. The metal brace stirrup is attached to the sole of the shoe, with medial and lateral metal uprights extending to either a leather or molded plastic calf lacer. The molded plastic calf lacer provides the additional benefit of axial offloading [31]. This type of brace requires the use of a separate foot orthosis inside the shoe. Although not as readily accepted as the molded AFO, the metal brace carries less risk of skin breakdown, because there simply is less contact with the skin.

The CROW is a molded plastic bivalve brace with a walking sole attached. The CROW is made of molded thermoplastic and lined with a thick, soft layer of polyethylene foam. At a point in the healing process it can replace the total contact cast used to heal ulcers and fractures [35]. It typically is not a long-term bracing option. Ideally, the patient will wean out of the CROW and into an appropriate shoe with a molded plastic inside or a metal brace attached externally.

Shoe modifications

The sole of a shoe can be modified in a variety of ways for any number of reasons. Typically, shoes are modified for one or more of the following reasons:

- To replace lost motion
- To restore lost function
- To increase stability
- To aid in forward propulsion or make ambulation more efficient
- To offload areas of high pressure
- To help the shoe better fit the foot
- To accommodate or enhance the function of an AFO

Some of the more common shoe modifications will be reviewed in this section. They include rocker sole, extended shank, flare, and relast.

Rocker soles

One of the most commonly prescribed shoe modifications is the rocker sole. As its name suggests, the primary function of a rocker sole is to rock the foot from heel strike to toe-off without requiring the shoe or foot to bend. There are six types of rocker soles; the actual shape and type of rocker depends the desired effect and the individual patient's foot problem. In general terms, the biomechanical effects of rocker soles are restoring lost motion in the foot and ankle caused by pain, deformity, stiffness, or surgical fusion, resulting in an overall improvement in gait and offloading plantar pressure on some part of the foot [36]. All six types of rocker soles can offload the forefoot, which is beneficial and can help prevent ulcers as diabetics with neuropathy experience increased pressure under the forefoot [26,37]. In fact, the rocker is considered the most effective way to offload the forefoot [38].

There are two terms that need explanation to discuss rocker soles: (1) the *midstance*, or the section of the rocker sole that is in contact with the ground when standing erect and (2) the *apex*, or high point, of the rocker sole located at the distal end of the midstance [29]. These terms are illustrated in Fig. 4. Proper placement of the apex is critical to the success of the modification. The apex should be placed just proximal to any area for which pressure relief is desired. For example, if the desire were to offload the ball of the foot, the apex would be placed directly behind the metatarsal heads.

Many off-the-shelf walking shoes and running shoes are built with a mild rocker sole. This simple, generic rocker often is adequate for a foot that is not at risk. It provides some metatarsal head relief and gait assistance; however, for the patient who requires more relief or has deformity or neuropathy, a custom rocker sole is indicated. An explanation of the six types of rocker soles follows [15,29]:

- Mild rocker sole—This is the most widely used rocker sole. Using a mild rock at the heel and at the toe, it can relieve mild metatarsal pressure and can assist in gait by increasing forward propulsion. The other types of rocker soles essentially are variations on this basic rocker (Fig. 5A).
- Heel-to-toe rocker sole—This type of sole is shaped with a more accentuated rocker angle at both the heel and toe. It is intended to dramatically increase propulsion at toe-off, decrease pressure on heel strike, and reduce the need for ankle motion. This modification may be indicated for patients that have had an ankle or subtalar joint fusion, fixed claw or hammertoe deformities, midfoot amputation, or calcaneal ulcers (Fig. 5B).
- Toe-only rocker sole—The toe-only rocker has no heel rock, only a rocker angle at the front with the midstance extending all the way to the back of the heel. This rocker is designed to increase weight bearing proximal to the metatarsal heads, provide a stable midstance, and reduce the need for toe dorsiflexion. It is useful for addressing forefoot

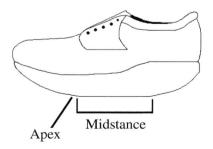

Fig. 4. Proper placement of the apex and midstance of a rocker sole.

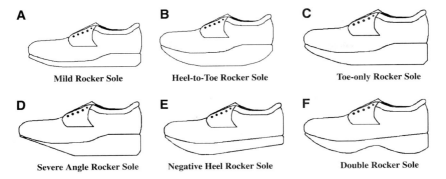

Fig. 5. (*A–F*) The six different types of rocker soles.

issues in a patient who experiences difficulties with stability or proprioception (Fig. 5C).

- Severe angle rocker sole—As the name suggests, this rocker sole has a much more severe angle at the toe than the toe-only rocker sole. It has no heel rocker angle. This rocker sole significantly reduces weight-bearing pressures distal to the ball of the foot and is therefore indicated for extreme relief of metatarsal head or toe-tip ulcerations (Fig. 5D).
- Negative heel rocker sole—The negative heel rocker is shaped with a rocker angle at the toe, with the heel height actually lower than the height of the sole under the ball of the foot. The purpose of this rocker sole is to accommodate a foot fixed in dorsiflexion or to relieve forefoot pressures by shifting them to the midfoot and heel. Because the effect is achieved in part by lowering the heel height, the height of the sole can be minimized, whereas other types of rockers may require the addition of material to the factory sole. This modification is contraindicated for persons with balance or proprioception deficiencies or the inability to attain the necessary ankle dorsiflexion because of arthritis, fusion, or tendoachilles contracture (Fig. 5E).
- Double rocker sole—This type of rocker sole actually consists of two shorter rocker soles with two short midstances. It is used to treat midfoot pathology. An unmodified shoe and shoes with the other types of rocker soles actually increase pressure under the midfoot (when compared with barefoot), but the double rocker sole does not [37]. This modification can be used to offload midfoot prominences such as those associated with a Charcot foot deformity (Fig. 5F).

Extended shank

The extended shank is made of either spring steel or carbon graphite composite. It is inserted between the layers of the sole, extending from the heel to the toe of the shoe. The carbon fiber shank is lighter than the spring steel shank, but it susceptible to breakage when subjected to extreme repetitive forces, such as being used in the sole of a shoe to which a dorsiflexion-stop brace has been attached and is being used by a very large person.

It is used commonly in conjunction with a rocker sole and in fact can make the rocker sole more effective. The shank keeps the shoe from bending, thus reducing forces through the midfoot and forefoot. It strengthens the entire sole and shoe and maintains the continuity of the rocker sole [9]. A useful application of the extended shank is to replace the lever arm that is lost when the great toe of entire forefoot has been amputated. It is also indicated for hallux limitus or rigidus and limited ankle motion. It also can be used to splint and protect the midfoot from bending stresses in a Charcot foot.

Flares

The flare acts as an outrigger, adding to the stability of the shoe and the foot. A flare is a strip of firm material added to either the medial or lateral side of the shoe—or both. The purpose is to increase medial/lateral stability and provide a wider base of support for the foot [39]. It can be helpful for a patient who has had a partial foot amputation or has a fixed varus or valgus ankle deformity.

Relast

Many off-the-shelf shoes can be relasted to accommodate severe deformities [39]. As discussed previously, custom shoes can be very expensive, and patients often are not receptive to the idea of wearing them. Relasting is a viable alternative to custom shoes for many patients.

This process involves customizing an off-the-shelf shoe by widening it through the midfoot or forefoot, to fit a foot that would otherwise not be able to use an off-the-shelf shoe. This is achieved by removing the outsole and making a cut through the sole, midsole, and innersole and widening the shoe according to a pattern of the foot. A new outsole is applied, and to the casual observer the shoe looks "normal."

Relasting a shoe may be indicated for a severe rigid pes planus deformity or a midfoot that has widened owing to Charcot arthropathy.

Summary

Research as well as clinical experience has shown that pedorthic and orthotic modalities can be valuable tools in the care of the diabetic foot. The team approach is probably more beneficial to the successful treatment of the diabetic foot than nearly any other problem the physician encounters. Understanding pedorthic and orthotic principles and how to include and use the appropriate clinicians on the team can simplify the patient care process while decreasing complications such as ulcerations and amputations.

References

[1] Bild DE, Selby JV, Sinnock Browner WS, et al. Lower-extremity amputations in people with diabetes: epidemiology and prevention. Diabetes Care 1989;1:24–31.

[2] Hunt C. Preventing foot problems in diabetic patients. AJN 1996;5:16EE–16HH.

[3] Levin ME. Preventing amputation in the patient with diabetes. Diabetes Care 1995;10:1390.

[4] Mayfield JA, Reiber GS, Sanders LJ, et al. Preventive foot care in people with diabetes. Diabetes Care 2002;25:569–70.

[5] American Podiatric Medicine Association. "Diabetes and Your Feet" Harris Interactive On-line Survey. Press release, April 8, 2002.

[6] Coleman WC. Footwear for injury prevention: correlation with risk category. In: Levin ME, O'Neal LW, Bowker JH, editors. The diabetic foot. 5th edition. St. Louis (MO): Mosby-Year Book; 1993. p. 437.

[7] Edmonds ME, Blundell MP, Morris ME, et al. Improved survival of the diabetic foot: the role of a specialized foot clinic. QJM 1986;60:763–71.

[8] Hobgood E. Conservative therapy of foot abnormalities, infections and vascular insufficiency. In: Davidson JK, editor. Clinical diabetes mellitus. New York: Thieme Publishers; 1986. p. 599–610.

[9] Janisse DJ. The role of the pedorthist in the prevention and management of diabetic foot ulcers. Ostomy Wound Manage 1994;8:54–65.

[10] Brodsky JW, Crenshaw SJ, Kirksey BS, et al. Eliminating the risk of foot ulcerations. Orthopedic Technology Review 2001;3:2.

[11] Pedorthic Footwear Association. Pedorthic reference guide. Columbia (MD): Pedorthic Footwear Association; 1996.

[12] Redford JB. Basic principles of orthotics and rehabilitation technology. In: Redford JB, Basmajian JV, Trautman P, editors. Orthotics: clinical practice and rehabilitation technology. Churchill Livingstone; 1995.

[13] Reiber GE, Smith DG, Wallace C, et al. Clinical trial of footwear in patients with diabetes. JAMA 2002;287(19).

[14] Sanders LJ. Diabetes mellitus: Prevention of amputation. J Am Podiatr Med Assoc 1994; 84(9):483.

[15] Janisse DJ. Prescription insoles and footwear. Clin Podiatr Med Surg 1995;1:41–61.

[16] Janisse DJ. Art and science of fitting shoes. Foot Ankle 1992;5:257–62.

[17] Rossi WA, Tennant R. Professional shoe fitting. New York: National Shoe Retailers Association; 1984.

[18] Rossi WA. The high incidence of mismated feet in the population. Foot Ankle 1983;4(2): 105–12.

[19] Frey C. Shoes. In: Goldberg B, Hsu J, editors. Atlas of orthoses and assistive devices. 3rd edition. St. Louis (MO): Mosby; 1997.

[20] Frey C, Thompson F, Smith J, et al. American Orthopedic Foot and Ankle Society women's shoe survey. Foot Ankle 1993;14(2):78–81.

[21] Michaud TC. Foot orthoses and other forms of conservative foot care. Newton (MA): Michaud; 1997.

[22] Chantelau E, Haage P. An audit of cushioned diabetic footwear: relation to patient compliance. Diabet Med 1993;10:114.

[23] Sinacore DR, Mueller MJ. Total contact casting in the treatment of neuropathic ulcers. In: Levin ME, O'Neal LW, Bowker JH, editors. The diabetic foot. 5th edition. St. Louis (MO): Mosby-Year Book; 1993. p. 283.

[24] Janisse DJ. A scientific approach to insole design for the diabetic foot. Foot 1993;3:105–8.

[25] Brodsky JW, Kourosh S, Stills M, et al. Objective evaluation of insert material for diabetic and athletic footwear. Foot Ankle 1988;9:111.

[26] Caselli A, Pham H, Giurini JM, et al. The forefoot-to-rearfoot plantar pressure ratio is increased in severe diabetic neuropathy and can predict ulceration. Diabetes Care 2002;25: 1066–71.

[27] Kuncir EJ, Wirta RW, Golbranson FL. Load-bearing characteristics of polyethylene foam: an examination of structural and compression properties. J Rehabil Res Dev 1990;27:229.

[28] Leber C, Evanski PM. A comparison of shoe insole materials in plantar pressure relief. Prosthet Orthot Int 1986;10:135.

[29] Janisse DJ. Pedorthic Care of the diabetic foot. In: Levin ME, O'Neal LW, Bowker JH, editors. The diabetic foot. 5th edition. St. Louis (MO): Mosby-Year Book; 1993. p. 549.

[30] Boulton AJ, Franks CI, Betts RP, et al. Reduction of abnormal foot pressure in diabetic neuropathy using a new polymer insole material. Diabetes Care 1984;7(1):42–6.

[31] Michael JW. Lower limb orthoses. In: Goldberg B, Hsu J, editors. Atlas of orthoses and assistive devices. 3rd edition. St. Louis (MO): Mosby; 1997. P. 209, 211, 214–6.

[32] Wu K. Foot orthoses: principles and clinical applications. Baltimore (MD): Williams & Wilkins; 1990.

[33] Trautman P. Lower limb orthoses. In: Redford JB, Basmajian JV, Trautman P, editors. Orthotics: clinical practice and rehabilitation technology. New York: Churchill Livingstone; 1995.

[34] Johnson JE, Geppert MJ. Prescription footwear. In: Sammarco GJ, Cooper PS, editors. Foot & ankle manual. 2nd edition. Baltimore (MD): Williams & Wilkins; 1998. p. 393.

[35] Sommer TC, Lee TH. Charcot foot: the diagnostic dilemma. Am Fam Physician 2001;64: 1591–8.

[36] Nawoczenski DA, Birke JA, Coleman WC. Effect of rocker sole design on plantar forefoot pressures. J Am Pod Med Assoc 1988;78:455–60.

[37] Janisse D, Brown D, Wertsch J, et al. Effects of rocker soles on plantar pressures and lower extremity biomechanics. Arch Phys Med Rehabil 2004;85:81–6.

[38] Praet SF, Louwerens JK. The influence of shoe design on plantar pressures in neuropathic feet. Diabetes Care 2003;26:441–5.

[39] Marzano R. Fabricating shoe modifications and foot orthoses. In: Janisse DJ, editor. Introduction to pedorthics. Columbia (MD): Pedorthic Footwear Association; 1998.

ELSEVIER
SAUNDERS

Foot Ankle Clin N Am
11 (2006) 735–743

FOOT AND
ANKLE CLINICS

Nonsurgical Strategies for Healing and Preventing Recurrence of Diabetic Foot Ulcers

Peter R. Cavanagh, PhD, DSc[a,b,c,d,*],
Tammy M. Owings, MS[a]

[a]Department of Biomedical Engineering, Lerner Research Institute, Cleveland Clinic,
9500 Euclid Ave., Cleveland, OH 44195, USA
[b]Department of Orthopaedic Surgery and the Orthopaedic Research Center, Cleveland Clinic,
9500 Euclid Ave., Cleveland, OH 44195, USA
[c]Diabetic Foot Care Program, Cleveland Clinic, 9500 Euclid Ave., Cleveland, OH 44195, USA
[d]Department of Molecular Medicine, Cleveland Clinic Lerner College of Medicine of Case
Western Reserve University, Cleveland, OH, USA

Orthopedic surgeons can find the management of typical plantar diabetic foot ulcers problematic because ulcer healing does not always require surgical intervention and because ulcers sometimes seem unresponsive to conservative treatment. Even in cases in which healing is achieved, the same patients seem to return again and again with ulcers at the same or different sites. Many new approaches to wound healing have become available over the last decade, such as bioengineered skin equivalents [1] and topical growth factors [2]. More recently, the topical application of bone marrow–derived stem cells also has been explored [3]. Nevertheless, the use of these agents has not resulted in the dramatic improvements in healing for which many observers had hoped. Furthermore, the results of attempts at healing foot ulcers using "standard care" in the United States have been rather poor [4,5]. After a brief discussion of cause assessment, we examine

The corresponding author's work on the diabetic foot is supported by Grant Nos. 5R01 HD037433, 2 R44 DK059074, and 2 R44 DK62547-02 from the National Institutes of Health.

The corresponding author has an equity interest in DIApedia LLC (www.diapedia.com) and is the coinventor on US patents relating to a load-relieving dressing for wound healing of the ulcerated diabetic foot.

* Corresponding author. Department of Biomedical Engineering, Cleveland Clinic, 9500 Euclid Ave., Cleveland, OH 44195.

E-mail address: cavanap@ccf.org (P.R. Cavanagh).

some reasons for poor foot-ulcer healing and discuss a number of approaches that can be taken to enhance healing and minimize ulcer recurrence.

Assessing ulcer cause

Intake screening of ulcer patients should always include an assessment of peripheral sensation and vascular status to classify the cause of the ulcer as either neuropathic or vascular. To assess neuropathy, the 10-g monofilament test has emerged as the test of choice in an office setting because of its ease of use. There is, however, some indication that monofilaments from different manufacturers may give different results [6] and that a given monofilament may degrade with use. The most common initial approach to vascular assessment is palpation of pedal pulses, but this approach can be highly variable and inaccurate, particularly in patients with suspected lower limb arterial disease [7]. The ankle–brachial index, based on data collected using a handheld Doppler device, is a preferable approach; in addition to its utility for the identification of peripheral arterial disease, it also has been shown to be predictive of cardiovascular disease [8]. Because of false-negative results in the presence of arterial calcification [8], the measurement of absolute toe pressures or the toe–brachial index has been found to be more effective, particularly in patients with peripheral neuropathy [9]. The width of the toe cuff has, however, been found to have a significant influence on the result [10].

The results of a cause assessment will be useful in determining the need for referral in the case of vascular insufficiency, as well as in posttreatment planning for a primarily neuropathic ulcer. If a neuropathic ulcer was caused by repetitive stress, then either the footwear was inadequate or the patient was not compliant with prescription footwear or foot care instructions [11]. An assessment of cause can also influence treatment. For example, plantar ulcers on the hallux of a neuropathic foot are invariably the result of limited joint mobility in the first metatarso-phalangeal joint, which may need surgical attention or rigid-soled footwear.

Wound classification and assessment

Many schemes for ulcer classification have been proposed in an attempt to enhance the traditionally used Wagner-Meggitt classification [12]. These include the University of Texas system [13], the S(AD) SAD classification [14], the "PEDIS" classification from the International Working Group on the Diabetic Foot [15], and the guidelines of the Infectious Diseases Society of America [16]. The common element in these various systems is an attempt to characterize or measure the size or depth of the wound and presence or absence of infection. Although none of the classification schemes have found widespread acceptance, the current authors believe that the PEDIS system, which measures Perfusion (arterial supply), Extent (area), Depth, Infection, and Sensation, can be applied easily and can be useful for communication between clinicians.

The detection of osteomyelitis in the diabetic foot remains a complex and controversial topic [17], particularly in the setting of possible Charcot neuroarthropathy. The validity of the "probe to bone" test has been questioned recently [18], and the dominant current view is that magnetic resonance imaging and bone biopsy are the preferred diagnostic approaches [17].

Wound treatments

There is a plethora of recommended wound-healing treatments in the literature, ranging from honey [19] to hyperbaric oxygen [20]. Falanga has provided a recent review of wound healing theory and practice [21]. The choice for the surgeon is complicated by the fact that there are few controlled studies of treatment efficacy and few incentives for manufacturers of wound care products or specialty providers of wound care to conduct comparative trials. The economic benefits to the providers of such treatments as hyperbaric oxygen therapy are clear, however, and it is likely that this motivation sometimes dominates over the available evidence in the choice of a wound-treatment modality. Recently, negative pressure wound therapy (NPWT) has come into widespread use, although there are only two studies in diabetic feet comparing this approach with "moist wound care" [22] and moist-saline gauze dressings [23]. McCallon et al. [23] selected 10 heterogeneous patients with diabetic foot wounds and assigned them randomly to NPWT or treatment with saline-moistened gauze dressings. They performed primary closures on four patients in the NPWT group but only two patients in the control group. The method of achieving and determining compliance with a "strict non–weight bearing" regimen was not specified. Their results, indicating faster healing with vacuum-assisted closure, are unlikely to be generalizable.

Armstrong and Lavery [22] performed a randomized, controlled multicenter 16-week trial of NPWT in 162 patients with complex wounds (mean area 20.7 cm^2) secondary to amputation. The control treatment was moist wound therapy using a variety of products, and the treatment group received NPWT using the "vacuum-assisted closure therapy system." An off-loading device was provided, but compliance with its use was not monitored. In the NPWT group, 43 of 77 patients achieved complete closure (median time to closure of 56 days) compared with 33 of 85 patients in the control group (median time to closure of 77 days). These are encouraging initial results for large, complex wounds, but the utility of NPWT for the more typical smaller plantar wounds in the diabetic foot remains to be demonstrated.

Off-loading healing wounds

Regardless of the wound treatment used, the need for mechanical off-loading of healing wounds is shown clearly by a review of studies using the total contact cast [24,25]. A meta-analysis of published studies in which total contact casts were used to heal neuropathic ulcers (Ulbrecht JS, unpublished data) has shown that the average time to heal 88% of 526 ulcers in 493 patients was 44 days (SD, 11 days). The average prior duration of the ulcers in these studies was 184 days, indicating that many ulcers that had probably been labeled "non-healing" were simply being poorly off-loaded. Midfoot ulcers at the location of a bony prominence are particularly difficult to unload; for these, the use of total contact casts with wound isolation [26] may improve healing times. Total contact casting certainly can result in new iatrogenic lesions [27,28], but frequent cast changes and monitoring by skilled personnel can minimize complications. Where such criteria cannot be met, other approaches are needed.

Removable devices are subject to patient compliance, which, in one study of cast walkers, has been shown to be extremely poor [29]; patients wore the required device for, on average, only 28% of their daily activity. Attention has therefore turned to ways in which the patient has no choice but to wear an off-loading device. One suggestion has been to wrap a few turns of fiberglass cast tape around a commercial brace [30], but primary attention must be given to the foot–footwear interface, because this is likely to be the most important characteristic of the device. Felted-foam dressings also can be effective in off-loading a wound [31], and this technique has been extended by building load relief into wound dressings [32]. Such dressings, with suitable footwear, are likely to be less restrictive to the daily life of the patient than a total contact cast. Approaches that rely on voluntary off-loading (eg, crutches, wheelchairs, or other assistive ambulatory devices) are unlikely to be successful in protecting the wound from mechanical load. Although some studies have reported successful healing in "half-shoes" that support only half of the plantar surface [33], these, again, require subject compliance. It is unlikely that satisfactory load relief can be obtained by simply modifying the insole or orthosis inside the patient's existing footwear or by an unmodified surgical shoe, and these interventions are not considered to meet the acceptable standard of care.

Posthealing management

Long-term follow-up for a foot-ulcer patient is often difficult in a busy orthopedic practice, and there may be a tendency for the surgeon to feel that ulcer healing represents "mission accomplished." Unfortunately, such an attitude may condemn the patient to ulcer recurrence, because one of the highest risk factors for a new ulcer is the history of a previous ulcer [34,35]. It has been suggested that the most important criterion of success is "ulcer-free survival" [36], which has been estimated variously at between 72% after 12 months [37] and 0% after 40 months [38].

The follow-up process must begin with a gradual transition from application of a healing device to use of definitive long-term therapeutic footwear. The prescription and manufacture of such footwear should begin well before complete healing has been achieved because, in many settings, there is often a considerable delay between ordering and dispensing shoes. The patient's own shoes in which he or she ulcerated are a good starting point because, if the ulcer was caused by footwear or repetitive stress, the old shoes can provide a baseline on which improvements must be made. Ill-fitting footwear has been implicated in the high percentage of ulcers and events leading to amputation [39–41], and thus the prescription of new shoes should be recognized as a high-risk event for the patient. In-shoe orthoses for diabetic patients should be accommodative and not corrective [42], because use of the latter implies that forces are being applied to alter foot biomechanics, and these forces may be damaging to the tissues of the foot.

Although foot shape is invariably used in the manufacture of an in-shoe orthoses—by taking a cast or foam impression of the patient's foot—ideally the plantar pressure distribution during walking should also be known and combined with shape in the manufacture of custom footwear. Shape is a necessary but not sufficient factor in engineering a definitive plantar interface, because shape alone does not allow the visualization of regions of high pressure that need to be unloaded.

One approach to this process that we are exploring is shown in Fig. 1. The foot shape is obtained from a computerized imaging device (see Fig. 1A) located in the practitioner's office and stored, together with patient information and prescribing physician's comments and preferences, in an online database. The patient then walks across a pressure-distribution platform while the computer captures information on the loading of the plantar aspect of the foot during gait (see Fig. 1B). All data collected from the patient are then downloaded in a single encrypted E-mail (compatible with guidelines of the Health Insurance Portability and Accountability Act) to a fabrication site at which computer algorithms are used to design custom metatarsal supports on a "virtual" insole to unload at-risk areas and transfer load to other regions (see Fig. 1C). The final insole is viewed on a computer screen and sent to a numerically controlled milling machine for fabrication (see Fig. 1D). This approach, now being experimentally validated, has the potential to overcome the current subjective, nonstandardized, and often trial-and-error methods of prescribing footwear.

The configuration of the shoe into which custom insoles are placed should be given careful consideration. It has been shown that many neuropathic patients, particularly women, wear shoes that are too narrow [43] and that both elderly and neuropathic patients have foot length-to-width ratios that make their feet too broad for standard-width shoes [44]. When additional pressure reduction is required beyond what the custom insole and a conventional

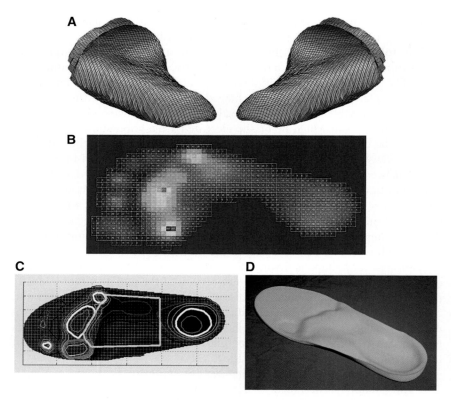

Fig. 1. A new approach to the prescription and manufacture of custom insoles. (*A*) Results of a digital scan of both feet. (*B*) Plantar pressure profile from a right foot contact during walking shows elevated pressure under the first, second, and fifth metatarsal heads (MTHs). (*C*) Shape (continuous color surface) and plantar pressure (contours) combined and trimmed to a shoe outline. The yellow leading edge is the basis for a metatarsal support designed to unload the high MTH pressures based on the measured plantar pressure contours. The "tail" of the intervention is smoothly and automatically merged into the foot shape. (*D*) The finished insole manufactured on a computer-controlled milling machine.

shoe can offer, rigid rocker or roller shoes should be considered. A number of studies investigating rigid rocker shoe designs have shown reductions of in-shoe plantar pressure under the forefoot of 20% to 50% [45]. Walking in rigid shoes does change the gait and can lead to instability, so care should be taken with patients who are already at high risk for falling.

Another important aspect of preventive care is regular visits to a foot care specialist. These visits need not be with the orthopedist, but they should be with a medical professional who can examine the feet for preulcers and remove excessive plantar callus. The importance of such preventive care has been highlighted by a study that found a relative risk of 11 for ulceration in patients who have plantar callus compared with those who do not [46].

Future developments

The clinical management of diabetic foot disease still lacks some basic tools that have the potential to improve outcomes significantly. In particular, most clinicians are not able to measure the degree to which a device unloads the healing ulcer or the success of a particular footwear prescription in transferring load from an at-risk area. Although such devices are available readily in the research laboratory [47], they remain cost prohibitive in a clinical setting. Even in the laboratory, the measurement of shear stress on the foot is still in its early stages [48], and shear stress may prove to be as important in the genesis of foot injury as the "normal stress" or pressure that is generally measured at present.

Summary

We have outlined an approach to the nonsurgical treatment of diabetic foot ulcers based on an understanding of their etiology. We have emphasized the importance of off-loading as the crucial element to success in healing foot ulcers and preventing their recurrence in those with diabetes. Computerized design of custom insoles can allow the unloading of elevated plantar pressure while incorporating the shape of the foot, which was formerly the major criterion used for insole design.

References

[1] Redekop WK, McDonnell J, Verboom P, et al. The cost effectiveness of Apligraf treatment of diabetic foot ulcers. Pharmacoeconomics 2003;21(16):1171–83.
[2] Smiell JM, Wieman TJ, Steed DL, et al. Efficacy and safety of becaplermin (recombinant human platelet-derived growth factor-BB) in patients with nonhealing, lower extremity diabetic ulcers: a combined analysis of four randomized studies. Wound Repair Regen 1999;7(5):335–46.
[3] Badiavas EV, Abedi M, Butmarc J, et al. Participation of bone marrow derived cells in cutaneous wound healing. J Cell Physiol 2003;196(2):245–50.
[4] Margolis DJ, Kantor J, Berlin JA. Healing of diabetic neuropathic foot ulcers receiving standard treatment. A meta-analysis. Diabetes Care 1999;22(5):692–5.
[5] Margolis DJ, Allen-Taylor L, Hoffstad O, et al. Healing diabetic neuropathic foot ulcers: are we getting better? Diabet Med 2005;22(2):172–6.
[6] Booth J, Young MJ. Differences in the performance of commercially available 10-g mono-filaments. Diabetes Care 2000;23(7):984–8.
[7] Lundin M, Wiksten JP, Perakyla T, et al. Distal pulse palpation: is it reliable? World J Surg 1999;23(3):252–5.
[8] Stein R, Hriljac I, Halperin JL, et al. Limitation of the resting ankle-brachial index in symptomatic patients with peripheral arterial disease. Vasc Med 2006;11(1):29–33.
[9] Williams D, Harding K, Price P. An evaluation of the efficacy of methods used in screening for lower-limb arterial disease in diabetes. Perspect Vasc Surg Endovasc Ther 2006;18(1):81.
[10] Pahlsson HI, Jorneskog G, Wahlberg E. The cuff width influences the toe blood pressure value. Vasa 2004;33(4):215–8.
[11] Knowles EA, Boulton AJ. Do people with diabetes wear their prescribed footwear? Diabet Med 1996;13(12):1064–8.

[12] Calhoun JH, Cantrell J, Cobos J, et al. Treatment of diabetic foot infections: Wagner classification, therapy, and outcome. Foot Ankle 1988;9(3):101–6.

[13] Oyibo SO, Jude EB, Tarawneh I, et al. A comparison of two diabetic foot ulcer classification systems: the Wagner and the University of Texas wound classification systems. Diabetes Care 2001;24(1):84–8.

[14] Treece KA, Macfarlane RM, Pound N, et al. Validation of a system of foot ulcer classification in diabetes mellitus. Diabet Med 2004;21(9):987–91.

[15] Schaper NC. Diabetic foot ulcer classification system for research purposes: a progress report on criteria for including patients in research studies. Diabetes Metab Res Rev 2004; 20(Suppl 1):590–5.

[16] Lipsky BA, Berendt AR, Deery HG2, et al. IDSA Guidelines: diagnosis and treatment of diabetic foot infections. Clin Infect Dis 2004;39(7):885–910.

[17] Berendt AR, Lipsky B. Is this bone infected or not? Differentiating neuro-osteoarthropathy from osteomyelitis in the diabetic foot. Curr Diab Rep 2004;4(6):424–9.

[18] Shone A, Burnside J, Chipchase S, et al. Probing the validity of the probe-to-bone test in the diagnosis of osteomyelitis of the foot in diabetes. Diabetes Care 2006;29(4):945.

[19] Molan PC. The evidence supporting the use of honey as a wound dressing. Int J Low Extrem Wounds 2006;5(1):40–54.

[20] Roeckl-Wiedmann I, Bennett M, Kranke P. Systematic review of hyperbaric oxygen in the management of chronic wounds. Br J Surg 2005;92(1):24–32.

[21] Falanga V. Wound healing and its impairment in the diabetic foot. Lancet 2005;366(9498): 1736–43.

[22] Armstrong DG, Lavery LA. Diabetic Foot Study Consortium. Negative pressure wound therapy after partial diabetic foot amputation: a multicentre, randomised controlled trial. Lancet 2005;366(9498):1704–10.

[23] McCallon SK, Knight CA, Valiulus JP, et al. Vacuum-assisted closure versus saline-moistened gauze in the healing of postoperative diabetic foot wounds. Ostomy Wound Manage 2000;46(8):28–32, 34.

[24] Mueller MJ, Diamond JE, Sinacore DR, et al. Total contact casting in treatment of diabetic plantar ulcers: controlled clinical trial. Diabetes Care 1989;12(6):384–8.

[25] Armstrong DG, Nguyen HC, Lavery LA, et al. Off-loading the diabetic foot wound: a randomized clinical trial. Diabetes Care 2001;24(6):1019–22.

[26] Petre M, Tokar P, Kostar D, et al. Revisiting the total contact cast: maximizing off-loading by wound isolation. Diabetes Care 2005;28(4):929–30.

[27] Guyton GP. An analysis of iatrogenic complications from the total contact cast. Foot Ankle Int 2005;26(11):903–7.

[28] Pizarro-Duhart G. Treatment of diabetic foot ulcers with total contact casts: a critical review of the current literature. J Wound Care 2005;14(10):465–70.

[29] Armstrong DG, Lavery LA, Kimbriel HR, et al. Activity patterns of patients with diabetic foot ulceration: patients with active ulceration may not adhere to a standard pressure off-loading regimen. Diabetes Care 2003;26(9):2595–7.

[30] Katz IA, Harlan A, Miranda-Palma B, et al. A randomized trial of two irremovable off-loading devices in the management of plantar neuropathic diabetic foot ulcers. Diabetes Care 2005;28(3):555–9.

[31] Zimny S, Schatz H, Pfohl U. The effects of applied felted foam on wound healing and healing times in the therapy of neuropathic diabetic foot ulcers. Diabet Med 2003;20(8): 622–5.

[32] van Schie K, Ulbrecht JS. Load relieving dressings. In: Boulton AJM, Cavanagh PR, Rayman G, editors. The diabetic foot. 4th edition. London: John Wiley; 2006.

[33] Chantelau E. Half-shoes for off-loading diabetic plantar ulcers. Diabetes Care 2001;24(11): 2016.

[34] Edmonds ME, Blundell MP, Morris ME, et al. Improved survival of the diabetic foot: the role of a specialized foot clinic. Q J Med 1986;60(232):763–71.

[35] Apelqvist J, Larsson J, Agardh CD. Long-term prognosis for diabetic patients with foot ulcers. J Intern Med 1993;233(6):485–91.
[36] Pound N, Chipchase S, Treece K, et al. Ulcer-free survival following management of foot ulcers in diabetes. Diabet Med 2005;22(10):1306–9.
[37] Uccioli L, Faglia E, Monticone G, et al. Manufactured shoes in the prevention of diabetic foot ulcers. Diabetes Care 1995;18(10):1376–7.
[38] Chantelau E, Kushner T, Spraul M. How effective is cushioned therapeutic footwear in protecting diabetic feet? A clinical study. Diabet Med 1990;7(4):355–9.
[39] Apelqvist J, Larsson J, Agardh CD. The influence of external precipitating factors and peripheral neuropathy on the development and outcome of diabetic foot ulcers. J Diabet Complications 1990;4(1):21–5.
[40] McGill M, Molyneaux L, Yue DK. Which diabetic patients should receive podiatry care? An objective analysis. Intern Med J 2005;35(8):451–6.
[41] Macfarlane RM, Jeffcoate WJ. Factors contributing to the presentation of diabetic foot ulcers. Diabet Med 1997;14(10):867–70.
[42] Cavanagh PR, Ulbrecht JS. Footwear for people with diabetes. In: Boulton AJM, Cavanagh PR, Rayman G, editors. The foot in diabetes. 4th edition. London: John Wiley; 2006.
[43] Reveal GT, Laughlin RT, Capecci P, et al. Foot and ankle survey in adults with diabetes mellitus. Foot Ankle Int 2001;22(9):739–43.
[44] Chantelau E, Gede A. Foot dimensions of elderly people with and without diabetes mellitus—a data basis for shoe design. Gerontology 2002;48(4):241–4.
[45] van Schie C, Ulbrecht JS, Becker MB, et al. Design criteria for rigid rocker shoes. Foot Ankle Int 2000;21(10):833–44.
[46] Murray HJ, Young MJ, Hollis S, et al. The association between callus formation, high pressures and neuropathy in diabetic foot ulceration. Diabet Med 1996;13(11):979–82.
[47] Bus SA, Ulbrecht JS, Cavanagh PR. Pressure relief and load redistribution by custom-made insoles in diabetic patients with neuropathy and foot deformity. Clin Biomech (Bristol, Avon) 2004;19(6):629–38.
[48] Mackey JR, Davis BL. Simultaneous shear and pressure sensor array for assessing pressure and shear at foot/ground interface. J Biomech 2005 Nov. 16; [Epub ahead of print].

ELSEVIER
SAUNDERS

Foot Ankle Clin N Am
11 (2006) 745–751

FOOT AND
ANKLE CLINICS

Wound Healing Agents

Samuel B. Adams, Jr, MD, Vani J. Sabesan, MD,
Mark E. Easley, MD*

*Division of Orthopaedic Surgery, Duke University Medical Center, Box 2950,
Durham, NC 27710, USA*

When not properly treated, wounds of the foot and ankle can be devastating for both the patient and physician. Therefore, it is important to recognize treatment options best suited for a particular wound, as well as the underlying factors involved in preventing a wound from healing.

The most common impediments to wound healing include wound hypoxia, infection, presence of debris and necrotic tissue, nutritional deficiencies, inhibitory medications, and metabolic disorders such as diabetes mellitus [1]. Only before minimization of these factors will wound healing agents be effective. Diabetes mellitus is a complex metabolic disorder that affects healing of wounds directly and indirectly. Specifically, diabetes causes alterations in microvasculature, nerve function, and the immune system.

There are a multitude of wound healing agents available, with some correlation to the type of wound or underlying disease, but for the most part the use of these agents is based on inherited common practice, personal preference, or marketing activities. Currently, the medical literature is replete of high-quality, randomized, controlled trials pertaining to wound healing agents, especially in the setting of diabetes mellitus. Therefore, it is the goal of this article to educate the orthopedic surgeon on the proper use of wound healing agents that can be applied to foot and ankle wounds.

Stages of wound healing

Wound healing occurs in three phases that are not distinct and separate but more a continuum of the entire process. The first phase or inflammatory phase begins immediately after the time of injury and lasts approximately 4 days.

---
* Corresponding author.
E-mail address: easle004@mc.duke.edu (M.E. Easley).

1083-7515/06/$ - see front matter © 2006 Elsevier Inc. All rights reserved.
doi:10.1016/j.fcl.2006.06.007

The initial goal of this phase is hemostasis and is performed through smooth muscle contraction and subsequent occlusion of the larger damaged blood vessels. The second goal of the inflammatory phase is the removal of bacteria, foreign debris, and other contaminants. Neutrophils migrate from surrounding microvasculature to accomplish this phase after which macrophages take over. Macrophages are the predominant cell in the second stage or proliferative stage of healing. Macrophages appear 48 hours after injury at the wound site to aggressively remove necrotic tissue and foreign debris in addition to initiating two important aspects of healing, angiogenesis and fibroplasia. The proliferative or fibroblastic phase can last weeks (approximately 3 to 21 days). The neovasculature, along with collagen and proteoglycan ground substance, form granulation tissue, which fills in wound defects and increases wound tensile strength between 5 and 15 days postinjury. This is followed by the process of re-epithelialization. A moist wound surface facilitates epithelial migration. The final phase of wound healing is the maturation or remodeling phase, which begins approximately 21 days postinjury and can continue up to 1 to 2 years. Remodeling is performed by collagenases that are secreted to help debulk and reorganize collagen bundles into a more parallel arrangement. With wound contraction, this produces an increase in wound tensile strength, which is maximal at the end of the maturation phase and 80% of the original uninjured tissue's strength.

Impediments to wound healing

As previously mentioned, there are several factors that can impede wound healing. Local tissue hypoxia is detrimental to all wound healing and may be the inciting event to chronic wounds, including diabetic foot and pressure ulcers [1]. Initially, hypoxia is beneficial to wound healing because it stimulates fibroblast proliferation and angiogenesis, but chronic hypoxia inhibits fibroblast replication and collagen production as well as predisposing the wound to bacterial invasion. Tobacco abuse, diabetes mellitus, peripheral vascular disease, and poor cardiac output are some of the concomitant factors that predispose a wound to tissue hypoxia.

A major impediment to wound healing is bacterial overgrowth. It has been reported that the number of bacteria needed to cause a wound infection is 10^5 bacteria per gram of tissue for most bacteria [2]. The mechanism of impairment of wound healing accomplished by bacteria is thought to be through the release of enzymes and metalloproteinases that degrade fibrin and inhibit growth factors [3]. Therefore, if infection is thought to be inhibiting wound healing, then debridement of bacteria and nonviable tissue should be undertaken. Debridement restores the host's natural balance of defense agents to bacteria, reduces the load of bacterial byproducts, and stimulates the production of local growth factors for healing.

Chronic diseases, as well as their medical therapies, can both significantly impede wound healing. Diabetes mellitus is a terrible disease that can predispose a surgical wound to poor healing potential or be the underlying etiology for the development of a foot ulcer. It is estimated that people with diabetes have a 12% to 25% lifetime risk of foot ulcer development [4]. Interventions such as glycemic control, ensuring adequate perfusion, and infection control are crucial to the management of diabetic patients with chronic wounds.

Nutritional deficiencies are also detrimental to wound healing. Serum albumin levels less than 2 g/dL have been associated with decreased wound healing from decreased fibroplasias, neovascularization, cell synthesis, and wound remodeling [1]. Additionally, it has been reported that after only 4 weeks of inadequate nutrition, phagocyte activity and lymphocyte function are diminished [5].

Wound healing agents

Impregnated gauze

Impregnated gauze are probably the most commonly used primary layer dressing on postsurgical and newly diagnosed wounds. They were developed at least as early as World War I to create a nonadherent barrier with variable occlusivity between the wound or incision and the rest of the dressing. Their ability to be nonadherent provides for increased patient comfort with dressing removal. They are composed typically of a fine mesh impregnated with a petrolatum emulsion or similar substance, as well as additives such as povidone-iodine, silver, bismuth, scarlet red, and aloe vera [6]. Adaptic (Johnson & Johnson Medical Inc., Arlington, Texas) is a commonly used dressing impregnated solely with petrolatum. It has an open mesh design that allows it to be completely nonocclusive. It therefore can be used on heavily draining wounds with an absorptive overlying layer, preventing maceration. Another commonly used impregnated dressing, but occlusive in nature, is Xeroform (Sparta Surgical Corp, Hayward, California). Xeroform has a petrolatum component but, in addition, has 3% bismuth tribromophenate, which acts as a mild astringent and deodorizer [7]. It should be used on wounds with minimal drainage, and is used typically as the initial layer on postoperative incisions. Additional applications include minimally draining graft sites and burns [7]. Betadine antiseptic gauze (The Purdue Frederick Company, Norwalk, Connecticut) is, as its name implies, impregnated with povidone-iodine solution instead of petrolatum. This dressing is used for contaminated or superficially infected wounds but should not be used on postoperative wounds as the cytotoxicity to new, fragile, or granulating tissue is well documented [7].

Other nonadherent dressings

It is important to briefly mention another type of nonadherent dressing that is used commonly but lacks petrolatum impregnation. These dressings are composed of two or more layers, one of which is a porous inner layer to allow exudate passage, and an outer layer that is absorbent [7]. They are best suited for weaping superficial wounds (ruptured bullae, abrasion, ulcers) to prevent maceration and allow the exudate to aid in adherence prevention, because they are not quite as nonadherent as petrolatum impregnated gauze. Examples of these dressings include Telfa (Kendall Health Care Products, Mansfield, Iowa) and Release (Johnson & Johnson Medical Inc.).

Hydrogels

Hydrogels are three-dimensional networks of hydrophilic polymers made from gelatin, polysaccharides, polyacrylamides, and sometimes other polymers [6]. These dressings come in the form of a gelatinous sheet or an amorphous wound filler [7]. The molecular nature of hydrogels allows them to retain fluid, allowing them to either absorb wound exudates or desorb chemical agents into the wound. Arguably, their ability to desorb is much greater than their ability to absorb, so these dressings should not be used on highly exudative wounds, because maceration may occur [7]. In fact, it is their ability to desorb saline or water that allows them to be used to hydrate desiccated eschars or dry skin. Hydrogels can be used on superficial acute or chronic wounds. Two examples of hydrogels include Curasol (Healthpoint Medical, Arlington, Texas) and DuoDerm Gel (ConvaTec, Skillman, New Jersey).

Hydrocolloids

Hydrocolloids are composite sheets of an adhesive inner layer, a hydrophilic polymer, and a water-resistant outer layer. They differ from hydrogels in that they are much more absorptive. The wound exudates interact with the hydrophilic polymer forming a gel that expands into the wound cavity. The increased volume of gel actually enables the hydrocolloid dressing to act as a pressure dressing. Thomas and colleagues [8] reported a 50% decrease in exudate production owing to the pressure dressing effect of hydrocolloids in venous stasis ulcers.

The composite structure of hydrocolloids allows them to be a complete and waterproof dressing. Patients may shower, and depending on the amount of exudate, the dressing can be changed every 1 to 7 days. [7] The occlusivity of these dressings makes them less than ideal for infected wounds. Hydrocolloids are best suited for mild to moderately draining wounds without signs of infection or wounds where autolytic debridement of necrotic tissue is desired [7].

Calcium alginate

Calcium alginates are naturally occurring mixed salts of alginic acid found in seaweed. They are fibrous in nature and come in various forms including ribbons, pads, and flat dressings, [9] allowing them to be used to pack various types of wounds. Like hydrocolloids, alginates function to absorb exudate. They form a gel as exudate is absorbed through a reaction of the sodium ions from the exudate and the calcium ions in the alginate [9]. The gel nature of alginates provides additional wound packing and a moist environment for wound healing, but these dressings do require additional overlying dressing material to keep the gelatinous mass at the wound. Alginates may be able to aid in infection control. Bowler and colleagues [10] in a simulated wound study, found that alginates effectively removed bacteria from the wound fluid by trapping them in the dense fibers and gel.

Silver

Silver in various forms has been used for medical purposes for thousands of years [11]. Traditionally, it has been used as a burn dressing, but more recently, newer silver dressings have crossed over into the general wound dressing arena. Silver has a broad range of antimicrobial activity against aerobes, anaerobes, gram-negative and positive bacteria, yeast, fungi, viruses, and even methicillin and vancomycin resistant *Staphylococcus aureus*. There are very few side effects from topical silver therapy; silver toxicity and argyrosis are the most severe, but these are reported to resolve with cessation of therapy [12]. Silver for dressing purposes comes in many forms, and the most common are creams and sheets. Flumazine (Smith & Nephew, Largo, Florida) and Silvazine (Smith & Nephew) are 1% silver sulphadiazine creams with the exception of Silvazine having the additional component of 0.2% chlorhexidine digluconate. Acticoat (Smith & Nephew) is a new nanocrystalline silver dressing available in sheet form. It is composed of the silver-coated mesh and a rayon/polyester core that helps maintain wound moisture. The nanocrystalline nature of the silver provides rapid and sustained release of silver to the wound. The Acticoat dressing must be kept moist with sterile water and can be changed every 3 to 7 days. Silver dressings are not complete dressings in themselves and usually require an additional layer to keep them localized to the wound. They are suited for a variety of wounds including burns and infected superficial ulcers. They would not be suited for heavily draining wounds, as maceration may occur.

Vacuum-assisted closure

Negative pressure vacuum techniques in the treatment of difficult wounds have been well described in the plastic surgery literature. The technique is designed to remove chronic edema and enhance localized blood flow to increase granulation tissue, which may expedite healing. Both retrospective and prospective studies have found improved wound healing and decreased length of time to full healing with negative pressure wound dressings. A study by Clare and Fitzgibbons [13] reviewed wound vacuum treatment in 17 diabetic patients with nonhealing wounds of the lower extremity, all of whom did not respond to previous treatments with serial wound debridements and dressing changes. Although many of these patients had previous surgical interventions including irrigation and debridements and amputations, 14 of these patients successfully healed their wounds in 8.2 weeks with wound vacuum therapy. From the patients who did not respond, investigators concluded that perhaps smaller forefoot wounds and large wounds in patients with severe peripheral vascular disease may be better treated by other modalities based on the three patients who did not respond in their study. Another study by Mendonca et al. [14] found similar results in patients with diabetic foot ulcers treated with wound vacuum therapy had satisfactory healing in 13 of 18 patients at an average of 2.5 months, and it decreased wound size from 7.41 cm^2 to 1.58 cm^2. A small, randomized, prospective review by Eginton and colleagues [15] found decrease in wound depth and volume for vacuum-treated large diabetic foot wounds compared with moist gauze dressings. Although more studies are needed to delineate appropriate patient selection for successful vacuum treatment as well and more data on results of vacuum therapy, initial reports appear to support vacuum therapy as an extremely useful healing agent for chronic foot wound or ulcers in patients with diabetes or peripheral vascular disease.

Hyperbaric oxygen therapy

Hyperbaric oxygen (HBO) therapy allows patients to breathe 100% oxygen in a chamber with increased barometric pressure. With enhanced oxygen delivery, increased arterial oxygen tensions provide an enhanced gradient for diffusion. Additionally HBO therapy decreases tissue edema. The high oxygen concentrations act as a direct vascular smooth muscle contractile stimulus causing arterial vasoconstriction. This may seem deleterious, but the high oxygen content of the blood compensates for any reduction in blood flow, and simultaneous increase in upstream arterial resistance in combination with decreased capillary hydrostatic pressures results in resorption of fluid and decreased tissue edema. Another beneficial effect of HBO is enhanced leukocyte function. Polymorphonuclear leukocytes generate oxidative bursts that are lethal to ingested bacteria and substrate limited by oxygen. Finally, with HBO therapy, there is a decrease in oxidate free radicals and mitigation of no-reflow process. Both in vitro and in vivo studies have found positive healing effects using HBO therapy.

Summary

This report presented a review of the process of wound healing as well as influencing factors in the process such as wound healing agents. A greater understanding of the alterations in diabetes mellitus allows selection of optimal wound healing agents to provide a more optimistic approach to wound closure for this large population of diabetics. We have reviewed some of the most common products used as adjuncts to the healing process. With newer innovations such as the use of negative pressure dressings and HBO therapy, the treatment of diabetic wounds continues to improve. With the increased number of wound healing agents, it is important to consider the type of wound and the conditions present when selecting one healing agent over another.

References

[1] Stadelmann WK, Digenis AG, Tobin GR. Impediments to wound healing. Am J Surg 1998; 176(Suppl 2A):39S–47S.

[2] Robson MC. Infection in the surgical patient: an imbalance in the normal equilibrium. Clin Plast Surg 1979;6:493–503.

[3] Robson MC, Senberg BD, Heggers JD. Wound healing alterations caused by bacteria. Clin Plast Surg 1990;3:485–92.

[4] Singh N, Armstrong DG, Lipsky BA. Preventing foot ulcers in patients with diabetes. JAMA 2005;293:217–28.

[5] Robson MC, Burns BF, Phillips LG. Wound repair: principles and applications. In: Ruberg RL, Smith DJ, editors. Plastic surgery: a core curriculum. St. Louis (MO): Mosby; 1994. p. 3–30.

[6] Ladin DA. Understanding dressings. Clin Plast Surg 1998;25(3):433–41.

[7] Hanna JR, Giacopelli JA. A review of wound healing and wound dressing products. J Foot Ankle Surg 1997;36(1):2–14.

[8] Thomas S, Fear M, Humphries J, et al. The effect of dressings on the production of exudates from venous leg ulcers. Wounds 1996;8:145–50.

[9] Pulman K. Dressings in the management of open surgical wounds. Br J Periop Nursing 2004; 14(8):354–60.

[10] Bowler PG, Jones SA, Davies BJ, et al. Infection control properties of some wound dressings. J Wound Care 1999;8(10):499–502.

[11] Dowsett C. An overview of Acticoat dressing in wound management. Br J Nurs 2003;12(19): S44–9.

[12] Hollinger MA. Toxicological apects of topical silver pharmaceuticals. Crit Rev Toxicol 1996;26:255–60.

[13] Clare MP, Fitzgibbons TC, McMullen ST, et al. Experience with the vacuum assisted closure negative pressure technique in the treatment of non-healing diabetic and dysvascular wounds. Foot Ankle Int 2002;23(10):896–901.

[14] Mendonca DA, Cosker T, Makwana NK. Vacuum-assisted closure to aid wound healing in foot and ankle surgery. Foot Ankle Int 2005;26(9):761–6.

[15] Eginton MT, Brown KR, Seabrook GR, et al. A prospective randomized evaluation of negative-pressure wound dressings for diabetic foot wounds. Ann Vasc Surg 2003;17(6): 645–9.

ELSEVIER
SAUNDERS

Foot Ankle Clin N Am
11 (2006) 753–774

FOOT AND
ANKLE CLINICS

Diabetic Neuropathy

Christopher Bibbo, DO, DPM[a,b,*],
Dipak V. Patel, MD, MSc Orth, MS, Orth[c]

[a]*Department of Orthopaedics, Marshfield Clinic, 1000 North Oak Avenue,
Marshfield, WI 54449, USA*
[b]*Department of Orthopedics & Rehabilitation,
University of Wisconsin Medical School, Madison, WI, USA*
[c]*Department of Orthopaedic Surgery, Veterans Affairs New Jersey Health Care System,
East Orange, NJ 07018, USA*

Most health care providers have been witness to the complications of diabetes mellitus imposed on patients suffering from this devastating disease. The basic pathoetiology of diabetes hinges on the improper metabolism of blood glucose, a ubiquitous fuel source for cellular metabolism. As such, diabetes imposes as a multisystem disorder, affecting nearly every organ system. However, the mechanisms involved in the specific manifestations of the disease (molecular pathology, cultural, genetic, lifestyle, and environment influences) are complex, all contributing in some way to the severity and development of complications in diabetes.

Aside from well-publicized celebrity patients afflicted with diabetes, many of us have had a personal experience with this disease and its complications, such as when a family member or close friend has been affected. It seems that every person knows someone with diabetes. So, how prevalent is diabetes? Diabetes continues to be a growing problem of epic proportions; 6% of the United States population is affected; 15% of the population over the age of 65 years is affected, with one third of new cases yet to be diagnosed [1]. This equates to more than 20 million Americans being affected by diabetes. These tremendous numbers speak not only of significant human suffering but also impart a sense of the staggering economic impact of diabetes to the United States health care system. In the United States alone, more than 100 billion dollars annually are spent (both direct and indirect) to address health care problems associated with diabetes [2]. This growing

* Corresponding author. Department of Orthopaedics, Marshfield Clinic, 1000 North Oak Avenue, Marshfield, WI 54449.
E-mail address: bibbo.christopher@marshfieldclinic.org (C. Bibbo).

epidemic presents serious repercussions on the lives of people, but it also affects those not suffering from diabetes, in that the economic burden of treating diabetes is passed down to every United States citizen.

The foot and ankle health care provider is asked very often to assess and manage foot and ankle complications associated with diabetes. The complications that we see tend to stem from two main organ systems affected by diabetes: the nervous system and the vascular system. The complications stemming from the nervous and vascular system are intimately intertwined. The same pathophysiology resulting in the development of neuropathy also results in the development of vasculopathy, which also contributes to the development of neuropathy. Why is the development of neuropathy so important? The answer lies in the fact that still, foot problems are the number one single reason for hospital admissions in patients with diabetes (approximately 20%). Among these foot problems, infections are still the most common reason for these hospital admissions. Foot infections are related directly to ulceration, which is linked directly to neuropathy. It has been well accepted that the annual incidence of foot ulcers in patients with diabetes in the United States is 5.6%; the lifetime incidence is approximately 15% to 25% [3].

Nonhealing ulcers precede 85% of diabetic amputations, with the majority of these ulcerations stemming from neuropathy [4]. This finding results in greater than 40,000 diabetic amputations per year, and it is believed that as many as 50% of these diabetic amputations are "preventable."

The authors find it absolutely amazing that in 2006, there is still an increasing trend in the number of cases of diabetes, and at times, it seems as though headway has not been made in preventing the complications of diabetes, namely ulceration, infection, and amputation. It is important for foot and ankle health care providers who treat patients with diabetes to have an understanding of how complex the biochemical and physiologic processes are and how these processes can lead to development of complications of diabetes, particularly neuropathy. In this report, anatomic and molecular pathogenesis of diabetic peripheral neuropathy is reported and current treatments and research are reviewed.

Pathogenesis of diabetic neuropathy

The underlying plot that sets the stage for the development of neuropathy in patients with diabetes is the same sentinel pathologic feature of diabetes: an excess burden of glucose resulting in metabolic instability. The clinical severity of complications of diabetes, including neuropathy is directly related to the severity and chronicity of abnormal glucose metabolism: longer and greater impaired glucose control results in more severe and irreversible neuronal changes. There are several key pathologic pathways associated with excessive blood glucose and the development of diabetic neuropathy, each biochemically complicated, but each interrelated (Fig. 1). From a molecular standpoint, the theme associating each pathologic pathway is neuronal oxidative stress from the production of reactive oxygen species (ROS).

Reactive oxygen species

To an extent, normal cellular homeostasis relies in part on the tight production and use of certain ROS: nitric oxide (NO), hydrogen peroxide (H_2O_2) and superoxide (O_2^-). During cellular metabolism, shuttling of electrons results in the production ROS, which are required for normal cell function. For example, cellular oxidative enzymes as well as mitochondrial electron transport (conversion of NADPH $\rightarrow$ NAD+) produces O_2^-, an important ROS in the cellular defense mechanisms used by the immune system. In the presence of excess glucose, the delicate balance of the production and management of ROS is disrupted; excess glucose results in the production of excess ROS. Similarly, nitric oxide (NO) pathway enters a perturbed metabolic state in the presence of excess glucose. NO is an ROS that plays a key role in cellular respiration and vascular endothelial vasodilatation and functions as an antioxidant and possibly as a neurotransmitter [5]. NO becomes a pro-oxidant when in the presence of O_2^- (such as that which occurs with hyperglycemia). Loss of normal NO function (induction of vascular endothelial relaxation) leads to a state of chronic microvascular vasoconstriction and nerve ischemia.

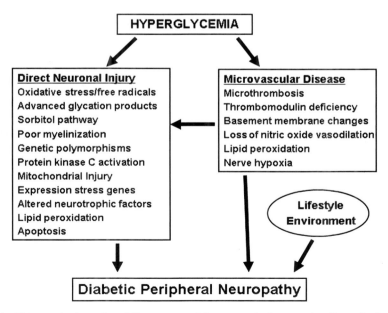

Fig. 1. The complex interplay of direct neuronal damage and microvascular disease in the contribution to diabetic neuropathy.

H_2O_2 is an ROS produced by several metabolic pathways or as the end product of the metabolism of O_2^- (eg, via superoxide dismutase). H_2O_2 is not without use, as it is a major weapon used by polymorphonuclear leucocytes. Normally, H_2O_2 levels are tightly regulated and it is normally inactivated ($\rightarrow H_2O$) by catalase (red cell catalase is responsible for the production of a bubbling foam when commercial H_2O_2 is poured onto blood); H_2O_2 also is inactivated by reduced glutathione and thioredoxin. Adequate cellular stores of reduced glutathione are critical to cell homeostasis, because it is used by an array of key reduction pathways, such as detoxifications. Excessive H_2O_2 levels (via hyperglycemia) help deplete cellular-reduced glutathione, resulting in a shift of H_2O_2 to the production of toxic hydroxyl radicals, thereby reducing the cell's detoxification capacity.

In the face of excess glucose, overproduction of ROS (beyond what is required for normal cellular function) results in the exposure of various proteins and cell membrane lipids (eg, mitochondria and the electron transport chain) to attack by ROS. Removal of lipid peroxidation products requires the use of cellular stores of reduced glutathione. Additionally, the accumulation of toxic peroxidation products is deleterious to nuclear material, resulting in increased apoptosis, decreased expression of anti-apoptotic proteins, and increased expression of proapoptotic proteins), DNA damage ($\rightarrow$ mutations), and a reduction in axonal transport. Additionally, ROS produced within the mitochondria is believed to render immediate nerve cell damage, even before excess glucose has been processed to alternative metabolic pathways [5].

Nonenzymatic glycosylation of proteins (production of advanced glycosylation end products), the polyol pathway, and the activation of protein kinase C

Under normal conditions, entry of glucose into the cell is controlled by insulin triggering a phosphatidylinositol-3'-kinase (PI-3 kinase)–mediated translocation of cell membrane glucose transport vesicles (GLUT4), which carry glucose across the plasma membrane, into the cell, and then directed to the correct metabolic pathway. This mechanism is particularly important for skeletal muscle use of glucose. In the absence of the insulin effect, an elevated blood glucose state develops; higher concentrations of glucose diffuse more easily across the cell membrane, accumulating in levels not required for normal cellular function. The excess intracellular glucose binds to cellular proteins (ie, enzymes, collagen) and acts as substrate for alternative metabolic pathways. In the process of nonenzymatic protein glycosylation, primary amino groups of proteins undergo nonenzymatic glycation to form Amadori products. Transition metals (which are poorly scavenged in diabetics) act as catalysts to take the Amadori products through a subsequent series of reactions to produce advanced glycosylation end products (AGEs), which are stable and irreversible. AGEs then bind to cellular receptors, proceed through a series of signaling events, using (depleting) cellular stores of reduced glutathione, reducing the cells detoxification power [5,6]. Clinically, measurement of AGEs in red blood cells (HbA1c) correlates with nerve dysfunction [7].

At the same time, excess glucose also becomes a substrate for aldose reductase (an enzyme that at lower glucose levels preferentially detoxifies aldehydes to inactive alcohols) with the conversion of glucose→sorbitol, an NADPH-dependent process. The reduction of glutathione to reduced glutathione is also NADPH-dependent; thus, a situation of competition for intracellular NADPH is created. The aldose reductase reaction requires reduced glutathione, further depleting precious cellular stores of reduced glutathione. Reduced glutathione is a critical cellular reducing agent used to neutralize hydroxyl radicals and prevent lipid peroxidation. Thus, any event that impairs the cell's ability to generate reduced glutathione places the cell in danger from attack by free radicals. Some diabetics possess a genetic polymorphism expressing a phenotype of two to three times normal levels of aldose reductase, increasing polyol pathway traffic. During this process, the cell shifts away from the production of myoinositol (an important component in myelin production), impairing nerve myelinization. Additionally, the presence of elevated sorbitol further initiates a cascade of cell injury by creating an osmotic effect, drawing free water into the cell, which is believed to be deleterious by initiating further oxidative stress, which, in turn, further stresses precarious stores of reducing equivalents [5].

In the presence of pro-oxidants (as described above), protein kinase C (PKC) becomes activated, whereas antioxidants inactivate PKC. The activation of PKC is noteworthy, because activation of PKC ultimately influences transcription factors that up-regulate the expression of genes that produce heat shock proteins and other kinases, which contribute to vascular atherosclerosis and apoptosis.

Nerve tissue factors

Proteins responsible for the overall health and maintenance of nerve tissue are termed *neurotrophic factors*. In particular, the nerve growth factor (NGF) and insulin-derived growth factor (IGF-1) effect a state of normal operating function in smaller sensory and autonomic fibers [7]. Neurotropin-3 (NT-3) is believed responsible for maintenance of large motor, vibratory sense, and proprioception nerve fibers. Diabetic rat models have shown delayed production of these nerve factors (eg, skin and muscle) in response to injury, as well as impaired retrograde axonal transport, rendering nerve tissue vulnerable after injury [8].

Reduced lipoprotein lipase activity

Lipoprotein lipase (LPL-ase) is a cellular enzyme responsible for the production of phospholipids from triglycerides and lipoproteins; phospholipids are major component of nerve myelin. In diabetic animal models, reduced LPL-ase capacity and subsequent defective nerve myelinization, both reversible by insulin administration, have been documented [9].

Nerve ion channels

Additionally, it is now thought that changes in nerve ion channels also may lead to nerve cell injury, contributing to decreases in conduction velocity (calcium ion cannels) and the pathologic propagation of pain impulses (sodium ion channels) [10,11].

Microvascular disease

A number of mechanisms contribute to diabetic microvascular disease. The resultant neuronal hypoxia contributes to the development of diabetic peripheral neuropathy. As outlined above, the production of AGEs leads to neuronal damage, but AGEs also damage the endothelium of vessels that accompany peripheral nerves. Oxidative stress-induced endothelial cell damage stimulates the production of the vascular endothelial cytokines, interleukin-1 (IL-1), tumor necrosis factor-alpha (TNF-α) and monocyte chemoattractant protein-1 (MCP-1). These cytokines induce the expression of the cell surface adhesion molecules vascular cell adhesion molecule-1 (VCAM-1) and intracellular adhesion molecule-1 (ICAM-1), which act as chemoattractants for neutrophils, resulting in microvascular inflammation. This process occurs in both endoneural cells and the vascular endothelium of the vasa nervorum [12]. The histologic changes associated with diabetic microvascular disease include microthrombosis and capillary obstruction associated with basement membrane thickening and duplication.

Interruption of the NO pathway is also an important contributor to nerve hypoxia. Very simply, NO (synthesized from the amino acid arginine via NO synthase) acts as a vasodilator. The ROS O_2^- reacts with NO, neutralizing the vasodilatory effect of NO, creating a relative vasoconstricted state; the reaction also yields the by product peroxynitrite, the degradation of which results in more ROS, namely OH− (hydroxyl radicals), further damaging the vascular endothelium. The diabetic neural microvascular bed also shows a significant reduction in thrombomodulin expression. Reduced thrombomodulin is believed to result in nerve microvascular ischemia by reducing the thrombomodulin-dependant protein C antithrombotic cascade [13].

The production of AGEs also elevates low-density lipoproteins (LDLs), which are associated with atherosclerosis. Coupled with changes (decreases) in NO, atherosclerotic vessels persist in a vasoconstricted state, affecting large and medium vessels as well as the vasa nervorum. Ischemia of the vasa nervorum results in nerve tissue injury and slowed conduction velocities [5]. Focal nerve hypoxia from arteriovenous (A-V) shunting may also contribute to nerve injury.

It is clear that the pathologic processes contributing to the development of diabetic peripheral neuropathy are complex and often interrelated.

Classifications of diabetic neuropathy and clinical manifestations

The majority of health care providers immediately think of sensory impairment in diabetes mellitus. Although sensory neuropathy often is the most common presentation to health care, there are several diabetic neuropathies, many of which do not involve the lower extremity specifically. In practical terms, foot and ankle surgeons are faced with problems arising from large fiber sensory neuropathy and small fiber polyneuropathies, many of which are painful mononeuropathies (including the motor neuropathies), and autonomic neuropathy (Box 1). Clinicians need to differentiate other causes of pain masquerading as neuropathy, such as plantar fasciitis, fracture, and ischemia. Other potential etiologies (nonhyperglycemic) for neuropathy in patients with diabetes include alcohol abuse, toxins, heavy metal poisoning, vitamin B_{12} deficiency, and monoclonal gammopathy [14]. However, the majority of patients seeking foot and ankle care suffer from sensorimotor and autonomic neuropathy, directly relayed to metabolic imbalance from their diabetes.

Large fiber sensory neuropathy

The most familiar form of diabetic neuropathy, large fiber sensory neuropathy, usually begins with a slow, progressive sensation of numbness, progressing symmetrically to loss of sensation. Loss of tendon reflexes and motor weakness may ensue. The progressive loss of sensation places patients at risk for ulceration. Clinically, when patients lose the ability to perceive a 10-g (Semmes-Weinstein 5.07 monofilament) force, they are considered to be at the threshold for loss of protective sensibility. Testing traditionally has focused on a global assessment of the entire foot. However, recent investigators have concluded that simple testing beneath the first MTPJ with a 4.5-g monofilament is accurate and reliable single test to determine loss of protective sensation in patients with diabetes mellitus [15].

Small fiber afferent neuropathy

Painful neuropathy is the hallmark of small fiber neuropathies. Motor function and tendon reflexes usually remain intact. Pain impulses are carried by myelinated A delta fibers, and even smaller and slower, unmyelinated C fibers. Along with loss of pinprick and temperature sensation, patients may experience varying degrees of pain, burning, and "electrical shocks," carried along the A delta fibers as well as deep (somatic) aching pain carried along C fibers. Inflammatory mediators such as histamine and prostaglandins (released by tissue damage) may further sensitize nociceptors. Additionally,

---

Box 1. Diabetic neuropathies and the subset of painful diabetic neuropathies

General diabetic neuropathies
Symmetric polyneuropathies:
- Acute sensorimotor polyneuropathy[a]
  Chronic sensorimotor polyneuropathy[a]
  Autonomic polyneuropathy[a]

Mononeuropathies:
- Cranial nerves III, VI, VII (ischemic)
- Thoracoabdominal
  Focal limb (*ex*-femoral)
  Proximal motor (amyotrophy)
- Inflammatory demyelinating

Painful diabetic neuropathies
Acute painful neuropathies:
- Distal sensory[a]
- Thoracic radiculopathy (ischemic)
- Lumbar nerve root/plexus (ischemic)
- Insulin neuritis

Chronic painful neuropathies:
- Small fiber distal[a]
- Large fiber distal[a]
- Compressive mononeuropathies[a]
  Carpal tunnel
  Ulnar (cubital tunnel)
  Common peroneal nerve[a]
- Proximal inflammatory demyelinating

---

[a] Neuropathy most frequently presenting to foot & ankle providers.

---

damaged axons show accumulation of sodium channels along the nerve, setting the stage for a relative environment for nerve hyperexcitability. Contributing to pain in diabetic neuropathy are ectopic discharges from uninjured neurons, N-methyl-D-aspartate (NMDA) receptor-mediated central spinal sensitization ("spinal windup"- continuous elevated excitability of central neuromembranes), and A-fiber sprouting with substance P neurotransmitter substitution ("spinal rewiring") [16].

Motor neuropathy

Motor neuropathy frequently accompanies established large fiber symmetric sensory neuropathy. Motor weakness compounds sensory loss, resulting in abnormal biomechanics, further placing patients at risk of ulcer-ation. Affected patients most often have involvement of the anterior and lat-eral compartments of the leg, involving the anterior tibial nerve and common peroneal nerve. The resultant weakness of dorsiflexion and ever-sion allows the overpowering posterior leg muscles to create an equinus. Wasting of intrinsic foot muscles creates claw toes, retraction of plantar fat pads, and exposure of metatarsal heads; the end result is forefoot ulcer-ation. Varus deformity may result when deep posterior foot invertors over-power weakened lateral foot evertors, with ensuing lateral column overload and ulceration. Compressive neuropathy of the common peroneal nerve and distal posterior tibial nerve may also develop.

Mononeuropathies

Diabetic vascular disease also affects the vasa nervorum of nerve roots and peripheral nerves (a form of "ischemic neuropathy"), resulting in deep pain, numbness, and motor weakness. When involving nerve roots, radiculopathic syndromes are mimicked; when peripheral nerves are in-volved, a compression neuropathy may result. Compounding this, almost one third of patients with diabetes exhibit a liability to compressive neurop-athies [17]. Management strategies, such as peripheral nerve releases, are thought to improve nerve function by release of focal compression and im-provements in local blood flow (vide infra). Diabetic amyotrophy often presents with similar clinical symptoms of pain and weakness but tends to result in more proximal (thigh) weakness acutely over several weeks, and im-proves over several months to years. Patients with overlap syndromes may show progressive weakness, with periods of exacerbation and fluctuating improvement, with return to baseline weakness.

Autonomic neuropathy

Autonomic neuropathy is well described for the cardiovascular and gas-trointestinal (GI) systems, affecting nearly one half of diabetic patients. Car-diac abnormalities such as arrhythmias contribute significantly to mortality in diabetes. GI dysmotility manifests throughout the GI tract, from the stomach to the large intestine. Neurogenic impotence is also a manifestation of autonomic neuropathy. In the lower extremity, autonomic dysregulation manifests in two major ways.

Dysregulation of skeletal blood flow is thought to be a major factor in the development of Charcot arthropathy and neuropathic fracture dislocations. Charcot arthropathy is a noninfectious destruction of bones and joints in patients with peripheral neuropathy, occurring in 0.5% to 2.5% of patients with diabetes. A current working theory for Charcot arthropathy starts with loss of sensation and position sense within lower extremity articulations. The lack of proprioception and sensation results in an abnormally elevated reactive force through the joints. The diabetic patient is at risk for reductions in bone mineral density not only by virtue of their peripheral sensory neuropathy [18], but also because of dysregulation of osseous blood flow (ie, increased periarticular blood flow), secondary to increased A-V shunting. The loss of joint proprioception and feedback allows abnormal forces to be directed through the articular surfaces and weakened subchondral bone. Subsequently, fracture and bone washout ensues, resulting in subchondral collapse and loss of normal bone architecture. In patients who maintain normal bone mineralization rather than acute fracture and washout, it is believed that joint dislocation occurs; continued weight bearing on dislocation may result in a bone fracture [19].

The first phase of the Charcot process is characterized radiographically as Eichenholtz stage 1 Charcot ("stage of development"), with bone fragmentation or joint subluxation–dislocation. Clinically, the foot and ankle are warm, swollen, and erythematous. The clinical appearance often is confused with an infectious process; a discriminating feature of the erythema in acute Charcot resolves with elevation, whereas erythema associated with infectious conditions does not resolve with limb elevation.

After the acute dysregulation, a reparative phase occurs as the body attempts to proceed through a process of organizing, absorbing, and remodeling the affected articulations. Typically, the reparative phase is limited and only allows for a partial reconstitution of bone morphology. Radiographically, this "stage of coalescence" (Eichenholtz stage 2) shows absorption of bone debris and bony sclerosis. Clinically, the limb temperature begins to normalize, with a matching decrease in erythema and edema. The "reparative phase" (Eichenholtz stage 3) is a continuum of stage 2, with further bony sclerosis, fusion, and rounding of large fragments, exuberant bone production, and evidence of joint immobility. Clinically, the foot temperature has normalized (matches contralateral limb) and acute mobile edema has resolved, but soft tissue is thickened and indurated. Mechanical stability may ensue, with or without bony prominence, or in contrast, mechanical instability and severe deformity may result. Thus, the end result of an acute Charcot process varies from simple collapse of an isolated joint to polyarticular destruction, dislocation, pulverization of bones, and severe limb instability (Fig. 2). In the face of osseous distortion, continued mechanical malalignment may result in further osseous destruction. Ulceration and infection may occur when an insensate patient begins to bear weight on a deformed or mechanically unstable limb.

More recently, a proposed mechanism for the development of acute Charcot suggests that an initial insult triggers the overexpression of TNF-α and IL-1β, which, in turn, leads to the expression of nuclear transcription factor κB (NF-κB) and its corresponding receptor activator, RANKL [20,21]. It has also been suggested that neuropathy alone may also lead to overexpression of RANKL [20]. The activation of NF-κB (via RANKL) induces the maturation of osteoclasts (osteoclastogenesis) with the overzealous resorption of bone ensuing [20].

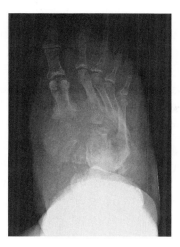

Fig. 2. Radiograph of Charcot midfoot. Note loss of recognizable midfoot architecture and soft tissue edema.

A strong association with increased early osteoclast and late osteoblast activity (elevated serum carboxyterminal telopeptide of type 1 collagen and procollagen carboxyterminal propeptide, respectively) in the Charcot process has been documented previously by Gough and colleagues [22]. This has called attention to the possible utility of TNF-α inhibitors and osteoclast inhibitors (eg, alendronate) in the treatment of acute Charcot arthropathy. However, factors controlling this process are likely multiple and inter-related, similar to the overall pathoetiology of diabetic neuropathy. A signal system responsible for termination of this process currently remains unknown.

A second manifestation of autonomic diabetic neuropathy is dysregulation of dermal blood flow and abnormal function of skin adnexae. Decreased production of protective essential fatty acids produces a dry, scaly skin that is prone to fissure and bacterial colonization. Surgeons caring for diabetics must recognize this condition and initiate treatment before embarking on surgery. Treatment includes skin conditioning with emollients, edema control, and efforts to decrease bacterial colonization (washing with chlorhexidine before surgery). Patients with lower extremity autonomic dysregulation may also have cutaneous venous engorgement as a sign of increased A-V shunting.

Treatment of diabetic neuropathy

It has been well established for years that tight glycemic control is critical to help prevent complications in diabetes, including diabetic neuropathy and microvascular complications [23,24]. The medical management of blood sugar homeostasis is beyond the scope of this report; therefore, attention is focused here on treating peripheral diabetic neuropathy.

Antioxidant therapy

Research has focused on several targeted therapies to prevent neuronal damage stemming from oxidative stress. To date, both aldose reductase inhibitors and nerve growth factor therapies have been met with limited success, although there are still ongoing aldose reductase inhibitor trials. Similarly, vitamins E and C have shown success in animal models by decreasing LDL peroxidation, but human studies have found uncertain value. Current research shows the most promise with the antioxidant, α-lipoic acid.

Alpha-lipoic acid

The ability of α-lipoic acid (also known as thioctic acid) to act both as a scavenger of ROS and a chelator of transition metals, has made it attractive as a potential therapy for diabetic neuropathy. Experimentally, Nagamatsu and coauthors [25] have found that α-lipoic acid can improve nerve glutathione levels, blood flow, and conduction velocities. Several clinical studies [26–30] have found that even short courses (3 weeks of α-lipoic acid, 600 mg daily) can improve symptoms and nerve function in patients with diabetic neuropathy. This has led to the current undertaking of large-scale randomized studies evaluating the efficacy and safety of α-lipoic acid for the treatment of diabetic neuropathy (NATHAN I & II trials), the early evaluation of which also appears to support the potential benefits of lipoic acid therapy for diabetic neuropathy [26].

Pharmacologic treatment: symptom-based management

The limited success of several preventative therapies and a lack of agents with current uniform treatment recommendations leave the everyday practicing clinician armed with treatment regimens that are geared essentially to address the symptoms of painful diabetic neuropathy. Currently, pharmacologic therapy for diabetic neuropathy is geared toward controlling the unpleasant symptoms of neuropathy. Several classes of drugs have been used to manage symptomatic diabetic neuropathy.

Antidepressants

The tricyclic antidepressants (TCAs) inhibit the re-uptake of norepinephrine (norepi) and serotonin (5HT). Norepi is believed to be involved with NMDA receptor-mediated hyperalgesia, and 5HT is also a mediator of analgesia. Currently, the most common TCA used for painful diabetic neuropathy is amitriptyline and, to a lesser extent, trimipramine. Dosing of amitriptyline is started easily at 25 mg daily and titrated to symptom relief and side effects. Bedtime dosing may help alleviate some complaints of unpleasant daytime side effects. Although electrocardiogram (EKG) monitoring is not uniformly recommended, we will obtain a baseline EKG reading (if baseline study not available within 1 year) in patients with a history of heart disease or when taking doses greater than 150 mg/day. Patients with known conduction defects should be referred to a cardiologist for consultation before treatment with TCAs or management deferred to a neurologist or internist. Patient compliance during TCA treatment for diabetic neuropathy may be limited by unpleasant anticholinergic side effects (dryness of mouth, dizziness, somnolence, urinary retention, blurring of vision, orthostatic hypotension, and EKG changes). These agents may be best suited for burning pain (versus deep aching and lancinating pain) [16,31]. In the authors' experience, the effective use of TCAs for painful diabetic neuropathy seems to be limited by a lack of coverage of global symptoms and TCA side effects.

Anticonvulsants

Gabapentin (Neurontin) and pregabalin (Lyrica)

Gabapentin and pregabalin are selective inhibitors of neuronal voltage-gated Ca^{+2} channels that contain alpha(2)delta-1 subunit [32]. Gabapentin has emerged as the initial drug of choice for treatment of painful diabetic neuropathy [33], with large randomized studies finding good tolerability, statistical improvements in pain scores, and secondary outcome measures of pain and quality of life [34]. Head to head comparison of the efficacy of gabapentin with amitriptyline for the treatment of painful diabetic neuropathy show greater improvement in pain, anesthesia, and greater tolerability of gabapentin [35]. When combined with morphine, a gabapentin/morphine regimen has been shown to achieve a better analgesia effect at a lower dose for each drug than either when used as a single agent [36]. Pregabalin has become an attractive alternate therapy, ostensibly owing to ease of dosing. A recent randomized, placebo-controlled study found that pregabalin 600 mg daily provided a statistically greater number of patients with improved pain scores and improved sleep [37].

Oxcarbazepine

A recent placebo-controlled study on a 16-week course of oxcarbazepine for moderate neuropathic pain yielded statistical improvement in visual analog scale (VAS), sleep, and global therapeutic effect. Side effects were mild and transitory [38].

Carbamazepine (Tegretol) and phenytoin (Dilantin)

Early studies on the use of carbamazepine found improvements in symptoms for patients with diabetic neuropathy. However, newer agents generally have supplanted the routine use of Carbamazepine [39,40].

Evidence to support the use phenytoin for painful diabetic neuropathy is poor. Likewise, newer agents have replaced Phenytoin, and its use is not routine. Thus, both carbamazepine and phenytoin are not recommended, and their use may be considered largely historical [41,42].

Topiramate

An anticonvulsant, topiramate, blocks kainite and glutamate receptors and voltage-dependant sodium channels, decreasing neuron excitability. Recent review of three double-blind, randomized studies yielded no statistical difference in topiramate-treated groups versus placebo and a 24% patient withdrawal rate owing to adverse drug effects [43]. Similarly, an open-label study on the safety and effectiveness of a 26-week course of topiramate for moderate to severe, painful diabetic neuropathy yielded improvement in worse pain symptoms, but a 40% patient drop-out rate developed, mainly because of adverse drug effects [44].

Opioids

Oxycodone

Controlled release oxycodone has been evaluated at doses up to 60 mg/d, with significant improvements in pain scores versus placebo [45,46].

Tramadol

Tramadol is an "atypical opiate analgesic" with low binding affinity to the μ-opiate receptor and inhibits the re-uptake of norepinephrine and serotonin. A randomized, double-blind, placebo-controlled, parallel-group study treating painful diabetic neuropathy found that, at a mean daily dose of 210 mg/d for 6 weeks, tramadol was significantly more effective than placebo. Tramadol-treated patients scored significantly better in physical and social functioning ratings; there was no significant improvement in sleep. A 15% dropout rate was noted. The most common adverse effects were constipation, nausea, and headache. Longer therapy (6 months) found sustained pain relief [47–49].

Selective serotonin reuptake inhibitors

Currently, limited data exist on the efficacy of paroxetine in diabetic neuropathy. Clinical studies on small numbers of patients suggest that there is some efficacy, but dosing may need to be titrated tightly to control symptoms. Serum monitoring may be required as doses escalate. Still, paroxetine is not as effective as the TCAs [50,51].

Selective norepinephrine and serotonin reuptake inhibitors

Duloxetine (Cymbalta) has been approved by the US Food and Drug Administration for the treatment of diabetic neuropathy, and few studies have reported on the use of duloxetine in the treatment of diabetic peripheral neuropathic pain [52–54]. Duloxetine is a balanced norepinephrine and serotonin reuptake inhibitor, mediating central pain transmission. One study has found up to 50% reduction in pain score versus placebo and less than 20% patient dropout rate during treatment [52]. Nausea is common and has been cited as the primary reason for discontinuation of duloxetine in trials [53]. Duloxetine should not be recommended as first-line therapy for diabetic neuropathy. The authors' limited experience with duloxetine has been patient noncompliance owing to severe nausea.

Inhibitors of Substance P

Topical capsaicin is a plant toxin derived from chili peppers. Capsaicin acts by depleting afferent neuronal substance P. Double-blind vehicle-controlled studies on topical 0.075% capsaicin (4 times per day) has been shown effective for reducing pain in diabetic neuropathy with subsequent improvement in daily activities [55–58]. Topically applied capsaicin has also been shown to be equally effective as amitriptyline for painful diabetic neuropathy, with fewer side effects [59]. Temporary burning or itching has been reported with the use of topical capsaicin. Although safe and effective, patient compliance is an issue with frequent applications, especially in patients who have difficulty reaching or seeing sites of application. Our experience is that unless highly motivated, many patients give up on capsaicin easily.

Anti-arrhythmics

The class1b anti-arrhythmic mexiletine has been used in the treatment of painful diabetic neuropathy. Mexiletine is a sodium channel blocker that acts by blocking neuron depolarization. Neurons with a low threshold for firing, namely regenerating fibers, are most easily affected. However, the therapeutic index for mexiletine is quite narrow: adverse effects include cardiac conduction blockade (contraindicated in heart block patients) as well as gastrointestinal symptoms, headache, and dizziness. Frequent EKG monitoring and early Holter monitoring is mandatory. Currently, mexiletine is not widely used. The authors do not recommend its routine use except when other agents are contraindicated.

Surgery for diabetic neuropathy

Pancreas transplant

Pancreatic transplant [60] or a combined pancreatic and renal transplant [61–64] has yielded stable metabolic state and improvements in patients with diabetic neuropathy. The degree of improvement in neuropathy after pancreas transplant is clearly linked to the premorbid state of the nerve; more advanced neuropathy will improve less compared with milder cases

---

Box 2. Other drugs and therapies on the horizon

1. Gene therapy. Murine models for gene transfer
   of vascular endothelial growth factor via herpes
   simplex virus (HSV) vector prevent loss of skin
   nerve fibers and reduce neurotransmitter markers
   (neuropeptide calcitonin gene-related peptide and substance
   P) associated with neuropathy [75]. The delivery of the
   neovascularization-inducing embryonic morphogen sonic
   hedgehog (SHh) has also been shown to induce vasculature in
   sciatic nerves in diabetic rats [76]. In a diabetic rat model,
   intramuscular injections of liposomal hemagglutinating virus
   of Japan (HVJ)/human hepatocyte growth factor (HGF) gene
   increased the density of endoneurial capillaries and improved
   nerve conduction velocity and the amplitude [77].
2. Protein kinase C beta inhibitor (ruboxistaurin). Phase II clinical
   data have shown that ruboxistaurin is well-tolerated and
   provides improvement in neuropathy symptom scores but
   provides no statistical improvement in vibratory threshold [78].
3. Substance P receptor Inhibition (NK-1 receptor antagonist).
   A recent randomized study found no improvement in
   neuropathic symptoms and objective parameters after
   a 2-week course of NK-1 receptor antagonist [79].
4. Acetyl-L-carnitine. Evaluation of the data from two
   randomized, 52-week treatment studies found improvements
   in pain, vibratory sense, and nerve fiber regeneration with the
   use of acetyl-L-carnitine in the treatment of painful diabetic
   neuropathy [80].
5. Monochromatic infrared energy (MIRE). A recent double-blind,
   placebo-controlled study found no improvement in perception
   of plantar sensation after a 4-week course of MIRE therapy
   [81].
6. Frequency-modulated electromagnetic neural stimulation
   (FREMS). A small, randomized, double-blind study (n = 31)
   resulted in significant daytime and nighttime improvements in
   VAS pain score after a 3-week course of FREMS, with benefits
   lasting as long as 4 months after cessation of treatment [82].
7. Electrical spinal cord stimulation (ESCS). Daousi and
   colleagues [83] assessed the efficacy and complication rate of
   ESCS implanted in eight patients who had severe, disabling,
   painful diabetic neuropathy for at least 1 year. Six of the eight
   patients were reviewed at a mean of 3.3 years
   postimplantation. Significant improvement in the background

pain levels and peak pain levels was seen. These investigators concluded that ESCS can continue to provide significant pain relief over a prolonged period with little associated morbidity. Stimulator-related complications were frequent but minor [83].

(younger patients, less duration of diabetes). Improvements in nerve conduction velocity occur over 1 to 2 years. Motor and sensory improvements may be expected at 12 months, and sensory improvements may continue thereafter. Improvements in autonomic neuropathy also occurs, but to a lesser degree than sensorimotor improvements. Nerve conduction velocity improves rapidly and then plateaus, whereas nerve amplitude may continue to improve over many years. Long-term follow-up studies show maintenance of improvement in neuropathy after pancreas transplant, whereas control group neuropathy continued to deteriorate. As one would expect, rejection of pancreas transplant results in a return to a premorbid state of neuropathy that occurs over approximately 1 year. Additional benefits have been documented after pancreas transplant, with major improvements in diabetic microvascular disease [65] and improvement in cardiovascular disease [66].

Peripheral nerve release

The natural question that foot and ankle surgeons will ponder: "is diabetic peripheral neuropathy preventable or treatable with surgery?" Both experimentally [67–69] and clinically [70], it has been shown that improvement in neuronal blood flow improves diabetic neuropathy by reversing nerve cell anoxia. Recovery of nerve function may also be enhanced by neurolysis (the release of a compressive neuropathy). The concept of peripheral nerve release as a primary modality to treat diabetic neuropathy was popularized by Dellon. The results of peripheral nerve release are encouraging [71–74]. Despite these positive reports, peripheral nerve release is still not a widely adopted technique to treat diabetic neuropathy. Publication of data examining the durability of improvement in nerve function after surgical release in a chronic, progressive metabolic disorder such as diabetes is awaited. It is likely, however, that in the future, further research on peripheral nerve release will better define a more specific subset of patients with diabetic peripheral neuropathy who, in conjunction with other standard treatment modalities, will benefit from early nerve release.

Other drugs and therapies on the horizon

A summary of other drugs and therapies on horizon are given in Box 2.

Summary

In this review, an in-depth anatomic and molecular pathogenesis of diabetic neuropathy is provided. Classifications and clinical manifestations of diabetic neuropathy are discussed. The current modalities of treatment and clinical research on this disorder are summarized.

References

[1] Sheehan MT. Current therapeutic options in type 2 diabetes mellitus: a practical approach. Clin Med Res 2003;1(3):173–4.
[2] Killilea T. Long-term consequences of type 2 diabetes mellitus: economic impact on society and managed care. Am J Manag Care 2002;8(16 Suppl):S441–9.
[3] Singh N, Armstrong DG, Lipsky BA. Preventing foot ulcers in patients with diabetes. JAMA 2005;293(2):217–28.
[4] Pecoraro RE, Reiber GE, Burgess EM. Pathways to diabetic limb amputation: basis for prevention. Diabetes Care 1990;13(5):513–21.
[5] Vincent AM, Russell JW, Low P, et al. Oxidative stress in the pathogenesis of diabetic neuropathy. Endocr Rev 2004;25(4):612–28.
[6] Cameron NE, Cotter MA. Effects of antioxidants on nerve and vascular dysfunction in experimental diabetes. Diabetes Res Clin Pract 1999;45(2–3):137–46.
[7] Podwall D, Gooch C. Diabetic neuropathy: clinical features, etiology, and therapy. Curr Neurol Neurosci Rep 2004;4(1):55–61.
[8] Brewster WJ, Fernyhough P, Diemel LT, et al. Diabetic neuropathy, nerve growth factor and other neurotrophic factors. Trends Neurosci 1994;17(8):321–5.
[9] Ferreira LD, Huey PU, Pulford BE, et al. Sciatic nerve lipoprotein lipase is reduced in streptozotocin-induced diabetes and corrected by insulin. Endocrinology 2002;143(4):1213–7.
[10] Hall KE, Liu J, Sima AA, et al. Impaired inhibitory G-protein function contributes to increased calcium currents in rats with diabetic neuropathy. J Neurophysiol 2001;86(2): 760–70.
[11] Shah BS, Gonzalez MI, Bramwell S, et al. Beta3, a novel auxiliary subunit for the voltage gated sodium channel is upregulated in sensory neurons following streptozocin induced diabetic neuropathy in rat. Neurosci Lett 2001;309(1):1–4.
[12] Siemionow M, Demir Y. Diabetic neuropathy: pathogenesis and treatment. J Reconstr Microsurg 2004;20(3):241–52.
[13] Hafer-Macko CE, Ivey FM, Gyure KA, et al. Thrombomodulin deficiency in human diabetic nerve microvasculature. Diabetes 2002;51(6):1957–63.
[14] Vinik A. Clinical review: use of antiepileptic drugs in the treatment of chronic painful diabetic neuropathy. J Clin Endocrinol Metab 2005;90(8):4936–45.
[15] Saltzman CL, Rashid R, Hayes A, et al. 4.5-gram monofilament sensation beneath both first metatarsal heads indicates protective foot sensation in diabetic patients. J Bone Joint Surg Am 2004;86–A(4):717–23.
[16] Spruce MC, Potter J, Coppini DV. The pathogenesis and management of painful diabetic neuropathy: a review. Diabet Med 2003;20(2):88–98.
[17] Dyck PJ, Kratz KM, Karnes JL, et al. The prevalence by staged severity of various types of diabetic neuropathy, retinopathy, and nephropathy in a population-based cohort: the Rochester Diabetic Neuropathy Study. Neurology 1993;43(4):817–24.
[18] Rix M, Andreassen H, Eskildsen P. Impact of peripheral neuropathy on bone density in patients with type 1 diabetes. Diabetes Care 1999;22(5):827–31.
[19] Herbst SA, Jones KB, Saltzman CL. Pattern of diabetic neuropathic arthropathy associated with the peripheral bone mineral density. J Bone Joint Surg Br 2004;86–B(3):378–83.

[20] Jeffcoate WJ, Game F, Cavanagh PR. The role of proinflammatory cytokines in the cause of neuropathic osteoarthropathy (acute Charcot foot) in diabetes. Lancet 2005;366(9502): 2058–61.

[21] Kon T, Cho TJ, Aizawa T, et al. Expression of osteoprotegerin, receptor activator of NF-kappaB ligand (osteoprotegerin ligand) and related proinflammatory cytokines during fracture healing. J Bone Miner Res 2001;16(6):1004–14.

[22] Gough A, Abraha H, Li F, et al. Measurement of markers of osteoclast and osteoblast activity in patients with acute and chronic diabetic Charcot neuroarthropathy. Diabet Med 1997;14(7):527–31.

[23] The effect of intensive treatment of diabetes on the development and progression of long-term complications in insulin-dependent diabetes mellitus. The Diabetes Control and Complications Trial Research Group. N Engl J Med 1993;329(14):977–86.

[24] Klein R, Klein BE, Moss SE. Relation of glycemic control to diabetic microvascular complications in diabetes mellitus. Ann Intern Med 1996;124(1 Pt 2):90–6.

[25] Nagamatsu M, Nickander KK, Schmelzer JD, et al. Lipoic acid improves nerve blood flow, reduces oxidative stress, and improves distal nerve conduction in experimental diabetic neuropathy. Diabetes Care 1995;18(8):1160–7.

[26] Reljanovic M, Reichel G, Rett K, et al. Treatment of diabetic polyneuropathy with the antioxidant thioctic acid (alpha-lipoic acid): a two year multicenter randomized double-blind placebo-controlled trial (ALADIN II). Alpha Lipoic Acid in Diabetic Neuropathy. Free Radic Res 1999;31(3):171–9.

[27] Ametov AS, Barinov A, Dyck PJ, et al. (SYDNEY Trial Study Group). The sensory symptoms of diabetic polyneuropathy are improved with alpha-lipoic acid: the SYDNEY trial. Diabetes Care 2003;26(3):770–6.

[28] Ziegler D, Nowak H, Kempler P, et al. Treatment of symptomatic diabetic polyneuropathy with the antioxidant alpha-lipoic acid: a meta-analysis. Diabet Med 2004;21(2):114–21.

[29] Hahm JR, Kim BJ, Kim KW. Clinical experience with thioctacid (thioctic acid) in the treatment of distal symmetric polyneuropathy in Korean diabetic patients. J Diabetes Complications 2004;18(2):79–85.

[30] Tankova T, Cherninkova S, Koev D. Treatment for diabetic mononeuropathy with alpha-lipoic acid. Int J Clin Pract 2005;59(6):645–50.

[31] Collins SL, Moore RA, McQuay HJ, et al. Antidepressants and anticonvulsants for diabetic neuropathy and postherpetic neuralgia: a quantitative systematic review. J Pain Symptom Manage 2000;20(6):449–58.

[32] Sills GJ. The mechanisms of action of gabapentin and pregabalin. Curr Opin Pharmacol 2006;6(1):108–13.

[33] Adriaensen H, Plaghki L, Mathieu C, et al. Critical review of oral drug treatments for diabetic neuropathic pain-clinical outcomes based on efficacy and safety data from placebo-controlled and direct comparative studies. Diabetes Metab Res Rev 2005;21(3):231–40.

[34] Backonja M, Beydoun A, Edwards KR, et al. Gabapentin for the symptomatic treatment of painful neuropathy in patients with diabetes mellitus: a randomized controlled trial. JAMA 1998;280(21):1831–6.

[35] Dallocchio C, Buffa C, Mazzarello P, et al. Gabapentin vs. amitriptyline in painful diabetic neuropathy: an open-label pilot study. J Pain Symptom Manage 2000;20(4):280–5.

[36] Gilron I, Bailey JM, Tu D, et al. Morphine, gabapentin, or their combination for neuropathic pain. N Engl J Med 2005;352(13):1324–34.

[37] Richter RW, Portenoy R, Sharma U, et al. Relief of painful diabetic peripheral neuropathy with pregabalin: a randomized, placebo-controlled trial. J Pain 2005;6(4):253–60.

[38] Dogra S, Beydoun S, Mazzola J, et al. Oxcarbazepine in painful diabetic neuropathy: a randomized, placebo-controlled study. Eur J Pain 2005;9(5):543–54.

[39] Rull JA, Quibrera R, Gonzalez-Millan H, et al. Symptomatic treatment of peripheral diabetic neuropathy with carbamazepine (Tegretol): double blind crossover trial. Diabetologia 1969;5(4):215–8.

[40] Chakrabarti AK, Samantaray SK. Diabetic peripheral neuropathy: nerve conduction studies before, during and after carbamazepine therapy. Aust N Z J Med 1976;6(6):565–8.

[41] Saudek CD, Werns S, Reidenberg MM. Phenytoin in the treatment of diabetic symmetrical polyneuropathy. Clin Pharmacol Ther 1977;22(2):196–9.

[42] Tremont-Lukats IW, Megeff C, Backonja MM. Anticonvulsants for neuropathic pain syndromes: mechanisms of action and place in therapy. Drugs 2000;60(5):1029–52.

[43] Thienel U, Neto W, Schwabe SK, et al. Topiramate Diabetic Neuropathic Pain Study Group. Topiramate in painful diabetic polyneuropathy: findings from three double-blind placebo-controlled trials. Acta Neurol Scand 2004;110(4):221–31.

[44] Raskin P, Donofrio PD, Rosenthal NR, et al. CAPSS-141 Study Group. Topiramate vs placebo in painful diabetic neuropathy: analgesic and metabolic effects. Neurology 2004;63(5): 865–73.

[45] Watson CP, Moulin D, Watt-Watson J, et al. Controlled-release oxycodone relieves neuropathic pain: a randomized controlled trial in painful diabetic neuropathy. Pain 2003; 105(1–2):71–8.

[46] Gimbel JS, Richards P, Portenoy RK. Controlled-release oxycodone for pain in diabetic neuropathy: a randomized controlled trial. Neurology 2003;60(6):927–34.

[47] Harati Y, Gooch C, Swenson M, et al. Double-blind randomized trial of tramadol for the treatment of the pain of diabetic neuropathy. Neurology 1998;50(6):1842–6.

[48] Harati Y, Gooch C, Swenson M, et al. Maintenance of the long-term effectiveness of tramadol in treatment of the pain of diabetic neuropathy. J Diabetes Complications 2000;14(2): 65–70.

[49] Sindrup SH, Andersen G, Madsen C, et al. Tramadol relieves pain and allodynia in polyneuropathy: a randomised, double-blind, controlled trial. Pain 1999;83(1):85–90.

[50] Sindrup SH, Gram LF, Brosen K, et al. The selective serotonin reuptake inhibitor paroxetine is effective in the treatment of diabetic neuropathy symptoms. Pain 1990;42(2):135–44.

[51] Sindrup SH, Grodum E, Gram LF, et al. Concentration-response relationship in paroxetine treatment of diabetic neuropathy symptoms: a patient-blinded dose-escalation study. Ther Drug Monit 1991;13(5):408–14.

[52] Goldstein DJ, Lu Y, Detke MJ, et al. Duloxetine vs placebo in patients with painful diabetic neuropathy. Pain 2005;116(1–2):109–18.

[53] Westanmo AD, Gayken J, Haight R. Duloxetine: a balanced and selective norepinephrine- and serotonin-reuptake inhibitor. Am J Health Syst Pharm 2005;62(23):2481–90.

[54] Raskin J, Pritchett YL, Wang F, et al. A double-blind, randomized multicenter trial comparing duloxetine with placebo in the management of diabetic peripheral neuropathic pain. Pain Med 2005;6(5):346–56.

[55] Treatment of painful diabetic neuropathy with topical capsaicin. A multicenter, double-blind, vehicle-controlled study. The Capsaicin Study Group. Arch Intern Med 1991; 151(11):2225–9.

[56] Scheffler NM, Sheitel PL, Lipton MN. Treatment of painful diabetic neuropathy with capsaicin 0.075%. J Am Podiatr Med Assoc 1991;81(6):288–93.

[57] Effect of treatment with capsaicin on daily activities of patients with painful diabetic neuropathy. Capsaicin Study Group. Diabetes Care 1992;15(2):159–65.

[58] Tandan R, Lewis GA, Krusinski PB, et al. Topical capsaicin in painful diabetic neuropathy. Controlled study with long-term follow-up. Diabetes Care 1992;15(1):8–14.

[59] Biesbroeck R, Bril V, Hollander P, et al. A double-blind comparison of topical capsaicin and oral amitriptyline in painful diabetic neuropathy. Adv Ther 1995;12(2):111–20.

[60] Kennedy WR, Navarro X, Goetz FC, et al. Effects of pancreatic transplantation on diabetic neuropathy. N Engl J Med 1990;322(15):1031–7.

[61] Muller-Felber W, Landgraf R, Wagner S, et al. Follow-up study of sensory-motor polyneuropathy in type 1 (insulin-dependent) diabetic subjects after simultaneous pancreas and kidney transplantation and after graft rejection. Diabetologia 1991;34(Suppl 1):S113–7.

[62] Muller-Felber W, Landgraf R, Scheuer R, et al. Diabetic neuropathy 3 years after successful pancreas and kidney transplantation. Diabetes 1993;42(10):1482–6.

[63] Allen RD, Al-Harbi IS, Morris JG, et al. Diabetic neuropathy after pancreas transplantation: determinants of recovery. Transplantation 1997;63(6):830–8.

[64] Tyden G, Bolinder J, Solders G, et al. Improved survival in patients with insulin-dependent diabetes mellitus and end-stage diabetic nephropathy 10 years after combined pancreas and kidney transplantation. Transplantation 1999;67(5):645–8.

[65] Abendroth D, Schmand J, Landgraf R, et al. Diabetic microangiopathy in type 1 (insulin-dependent) diabetic patients after successful pancreatic and kidney or solitary kidney transplantation. Diabetologia 1991;34(Suppl 1):S131–4.

[66] Jukema JW, Smets YF, van der Pijl JW, et al. Impact of simultaneous pancreas and kidney transplantation on progression of coronary atherosclerosis in patients with end-stage renal failure due to type 1 diabetes. Diabetes Care 2002;25(5):906–11.

[67] Low PA, Schmelzer JD, Ward KK, et al. Effect of hyperbaric oxygenation on normal and chronic streptozotocin diabetic peripheral nerves. Exp Neurol 1988;99(1):201–12.

[68] Smith WJ, Diemel LT, Leach RM, et al. Central hypoxaemia in rats provokes neurological defects similar to those seen in experimental diabetes mellitus: evidence for a partial role of endoneurial hypoxia in diabetic neuropathy. Neuroscience 1991;45(2):255–9.

[69] Hendriksen PH, Oey PL, Wieneke GH, et al. Hypoxic neuropathy versus diabetic neuropathy. An electrophysiological study in rats. J Neurol Sci 1992;110(1–2):99–106.

[70] Akbari CM, Gibbons GW, Habershaw GM, et al. The effect of arterial reconstruction on the natural history of diabetic neuropathy. Arch Surg 1997;132(2):148–52.

[71] Aszmann OC, Kress KM, Dellon AL. Results of decompression of peripheral nerves in diabetics: a prospective, blinded study. Plast Reconstr Surg 2000;106(4):816–22.

[72] Wood WA, Wood MA. Decompression of peripheral nerves for diabetic neuropathy in the lower extremity. J Foot Ankle Surg 2003;42(5):268–75.

[73] Rader AJ. Surgical decompression in lower-extremity diabetic peripheral neuropathy. Am Podiatr Med Assoc 2005;95(5):446–50.

[74] Valdivia JM, Dellon AL, Weinand ME, et al. Surgical treatment of peripheral neuropathy: outcomes from 100 consecutive decompressions. J Am Podiatr Med Assoc 2005;95(5):451–4.

[75] Chattopadhyay M, Krisky D, Wolfe D, et al. HSV-mediated gene transfer of vascular endothelial growth factor to dorsal root ganglia prevents diabetic neuropathy. Gene Ther 2005; 12(18):1377–84.

[76] Kusano KF, Allendoerfer KL, Munger W, et al. Sonic hedgehog induces arteriogenesis in diabetic vasa nervorum and restores function in diabetic neuropathy. Arterioscler Thromb Vasc Biol 2004;24(11):2102–7.

[77] Kato N, Nemoto K, Nakanishi K, et al. Nonviral gene transfer of human hepatocyte growth factor improves streptozotocin-induced diabetic neuropathy in rats. Diabetes 2005;54(3): 846–54.

[78] Vinik AI, Bril V, Kempler P, et al. the MBBQ Study Group. Treatment of symptomatic diabetic peripheral neuropathy with the protein kinase C beta-inhibitor ruboxistaurin mesylate during a 1-year, randomized, placebo-controlled, double-blind clinical trial. Clin Ther 2005; 27(8):1164–80.

[79] Sindrup SH, Graf A, Sfikas N. The NK(1)-receptor antagonist TKA731 in painful diabetic neuropathy: a randomised, controlled trial. Eur J Pain 2005;(Sep):28 [Epub].

[80] Sima AA, Calvani M, Mehra M, et al. Acetyl-L-Carnitine Study Group. Acetyl-L-carnitine improves pain, nerve regeneration, and vibratory perception in patients with chronic diabetic neuropathy: an analysis of two randomized placebo-controlled trials. Diabetes Care 2005; 28(1):89–94.

[81] Clifft JK, Kasser RJ, Newton TS, et al. The effect of monochromatic infrared energy on sensation in patients with diabetic peripheral neuropathy: a double-blind, placebo-controlled study. Diabetes Care 2005;28(12):2896–900.

[82] Bosi E, Conti M, Vermigli C, et al. Effectiveness of frequency-modulated electromagnetic neural stimulation in the treatment of painful diabetic neuropathy. Diabetologia 2005; 48(5):817–23.

[83] Daousi C, Benbow SJ, MacFarlane IA. Electrical spinal cord stimulation in the long-term treatment of chronic painful diabetic neuropathy. Diabet Med 2005;22(4):393–8.

ELSEVIER
SAUNDERS

Foot Ankle Clin N Am
11 (2006) 775–789

FOOT AND
ANKLE CLINICS

Osteomyelitis in the Diabetic Foot: Diagnosis and Management

Craig F. Shank, MD[a], Jonathan B. Feibel, MD[b],*

[a]Department of Orthopaedic Surgery, Mount Carmel Medical Center,
793 W. State Street, Columbus, OH 43222, USA
[b]The Cardinal Orthopaedic Institute, 259 Taylor Station Road, Columbus,
OH 43213, USA

Foot and ankle infections are among the most devastating and costly complications of diabetes mellitus. Foot infections are the most common reason for hospital admission for patients with diabetes mellitus in the United States [1] and are responsible for 59% of lower extremity amputations in these patients [2]. Caring for diabetes-related foot and ankle infections represents a huge financial burden to both individuals and society; the direct cost of healing an infection that required amputation exceeded $30,000 in one study [3].

Because of the difficult decision-making process involved, the poor long-term outcome, or perhaps the unpleasant nature of the infection itself, orthopedic surgeons often have very little enthusiasm for treating this complex problem. However, the rising prevalence of type 2 diabetes mellitus in Western countries assures that orthopedic surgeons increasingly will encounter patients with diabetic foot infections. Optimal care of the diabetic foot requires a multidisciplinary approach, and the orthopedic surgeon's knowledge of foot anatomy and biomechanics, surgical approaches and techniques, as well as footwear, orthoses, and prosthetics makes the orthopedist a critical member of the diabetic foot care team.

Often, the orthopedic surgeon is consulted to evaluate and manage the diabetic foot infection when osteomyelitis is found or suspected. Underlying bone infection is present in as many as 60% of infected diabetic ulcers [4,5] and was the most common clinical presentation of foot infection in one large series [6]. The evaluation and treatment of this common foot disorder is both difficult and controversial. This article reviews evidence and basic

* Corresponding author.
  E-mail address: doctorduke91@aol.com (J.B. Feibel).

1083-7515/06/$ - see front matter © 2006 Elsevier Inc. All rights reserved.
doi:10.1016/j.fcl.2006.06.008   *foot.theclinics.com*

principles regarding diagnosis and management of osteomyelitis of the foot in the diabetic patient.

Pathophysiology

The classic diabetes-related foot infection follows a loss in skin integrity of the lower extremity, usually a result of diabetic foot ulceration. Diabetic foot ulcers are believed to have a multifactorial etiology. Independent risk factors for ulceration include neuropathy, insulin use, foot deformity, reduced skin oxygenation, higher body weight, poor arterial perfusion, and poor vision [7]. Although inadequate blood supply traditionally has been considered the major factor predisposing diabetic patients to ulcer formation, neuropathy is now recognized as the central factor in the process of skin breakdown and is present in 80% of patients with foot disease [8,9]. The triad of neuropathy, minor foot trauma, and foot deformity exists in two thirds of patients with lower extremity ulcers [9].

Once the barrier of skin integrity has been breached, altered immune function may reduce the diabetic patient's ability to fight infection. Compared with a nondiabetic cohort, diabetic patients are at an 80% increased risk for cellulitis, a fourfold increased risk of osteomyelitis, and a twofold risk of both sepsis and death caused by infection [10]. A number of defects in leukocyte response and function have been seen in diabetic patients, including chemotaxis, adherence, phagocytosis, and intracellular killing [11]. Local wound conditions may be favorable for bacterial growth owing to slowed clearance of devitalized tissue and metabolic alterations such as hyperglycemia and acidic anaerobic products.

When a soft-tissue infection develops or bone is exposed to organisms colonizing an ulcer, bacteria penetrate cortical bone and gain access to the marrow cavity. Staphylococcal species adhere to bone matrix via high-affinity receptors for bone matrix proteins such as fibronectin [12]. Once established, bacteria can evade host defenses and antibiotics by hiding intracellularly, slowing their metabolic rate, or forming glycocalix biofilms. Bacterial antigens stimulate inflammatory cells to produce soluble factors (interleukin-1 [IL-1] and tumor necrosis factor [TNF]) which, in turn, stimulate osteoclast-mediated osteolysis [13]. In addition, bacteria have been shown in vitro to inhibit production of matrix proteins by human osteoblasts [14].

Microbiology

The most important characteristic of foot infection in the diabetic patient is that it is frequently polymicrobial. Ge et al. [15] surveyed the microbiologic profiles of infected diabetic foot ulcers (825 patients) and found that 75% of wounds had multiple organisms, with an average of 2.4 organisms per wound. Gram-positive aerobic bacteria such as *Staphylococcus aureus* and *Enterococcus faecalis,* dominated (68%), but gram-negative aerobes (24%,

Pseudomonas aeruginosa most common), anaerobes (6%), and fungal species (3%) were also present [15]. Like the overlying soft-tissue infection, osteomyelitis of the foot in diabetic patients is also a polymicrobial infection. Lavery and Sariaya [16] obtained more than one organism from bone specimens in 83% of patients, with an average of 2.25 pathogens per patient. *S aureus* and *Epidermidis, Enterococcus*, and *Streptococcus* species are most commonly isolated from bone infections. However, aerobic gram-negative rods and obligate anaerobes are also found in many cases. Because organisms involved in this disease are often found as contaminates in other types of infection, proper culture technique must be exercised to identify all organisms correctly. Special culture swabs and transport media designed for anaerobic (and possibly fungal) specimens should be used. Anaerobic organisms are more likely to be present in infections that are severe, long-standing, resistant to antibiotic therapy, or accompanied by necrotic material and a foul odor [8].

Cultures obtained from soft-tissue specimens do not reflect accurately the pathogens involved in underlying osteomyelitis. Superficial swab cultures from infected ulcers are notoriously inaccurate, identifying deep soft-tissue organisms in only 75% of cases and bone bacteria in only 30% [17]. In addition, surgically obtained, deep soft-tissue specimens do not correlate with bone specimens. Lavery and Sariaya [16]found that only 36% of soft-tissue cultures were completely accurate in identifying bone pathogens, even when samples were obtained during the same surgical procedure. As a result, the investigators recommend that physicians obtain both soft-tissue and bone specimens when cultures are used to guide therapy.

Multidrug-resistant organisms, particularly methicillin-resistant *S aureus* (MRSA), are becoming increasingly prevalent in a variety of infections, and diabetic foot infection is no exception [16]. Some investigators have suggested that this organism may be more virulent, lead to a worse outcome, or necessitate more aggressive intervention. However, there currently is little clinical evidence to support this conclusion, and three studies have found no difference in outcome between wounds colonized with or without MRSA [18–20].

Diagnosis

Clinical evaluation

Clinical evaluation of the diabetic patient with foot infection should be systematic and thorough. Basic principles for examining the diabetic foot should be followed, including inspection of the entire surface of both ankles and feet, monofilament testing to assess the severity of neuropathy, and examination of the vascular status of the lower extremity.

Foot infection in diabetic patients is most often a sequela of foot ulceration [21,22]. The site, size, and depth of ulceration should be documented. Ulcers that appear to be superficial can have hidden deeper components and should be probed for underlying bone or joint involvement, abscesses, sinus tracts, or extension along soft-tissue planes. The classification system developed by Wagner [23] is used widely to grade ulceration of the foot. Grade zero signifies an "at-risk foot" of a diabetic patient; there is no ulceration but risk factors such as previous ulcer, neuropathy, deformity, or callous formation exist. Grade one is a superficial ulcer without infection. Grade two is a deep ulcer exposing tendon or joint with or without soft-tissue infection; grade three ulcers have exposed bone, abscess formation, or osteomyelitis; and grades four and five are related to the extent of loss of vascularity of the foot, which can be either partial or complete [23]. Although ulcerations are colonized by local skin flora, this does not necessarily correlate with infection. In the well-perfused foot, the onset of soft-tissue infection is signaled inflammation. The infected part becomes red, tender, diffusely swollen, and warm. Fluctuance, purulent material, or a foul odor may be present. Granulation tissue appears less viable, and healing slows or halts. In the presence of ischemia, inflammatory changes often are reduced, but there is usually some evidence of inflammation or necrosis.

Although soft-tissue infections often are clinically obvious, the diagnosis of osteomyelitis in conjunction with diabetic foot ulcers can be very difficult. Systemic signs, such as fever, chills, leukocytosis, and malaise are unusual or late findings in foot infections, including those with osteomyelitis. These systemic signs should alert the physician to the possibility of a more serious or life-threatening infection [22,24]. During physical examination, signs of inflammation may be absent in up to two thirds of ulcers with histopathologic evidence of osteomyelitis [4]. Even when signs and symptoms of inflammation are present, osteomyelitis remains difficult to distinguish clinically from isolated soft-tissue infection or neuropathic osteoarthropathy.

Two clinical findings have been shown to help predict the presence of osteomyelitis. Newman et al. [4] found that the larger and deeper the skin ulceration, the more likely underlying osteomyelitis exists. An ulcer area greater than 2 cm^2 had a sensitivity of 56% and specificity of 92% for diagnosing osteomyelitis in their patient population. Deeper ulcers were much more likely than more superficial ulcers to overlie bone infection [4]. In addition to the size and depth of the lesion, the presence of bone within the infected diabetic ulcer is predictive of osteomyelitis. An ulcer with overtly exposed bone or discharge of bony fragments indicates a very high probability of osteomyelitis [4,5]. Furthermore, Grayson and colleagues [5] found that bone hidden in the depth of a diabetic ulcer correlates with bone infection. In their prospective study of hospitalized patients with diabetic foot infections, when bone could be palpated with the tip of a sterile probe inserted into the wound, osteomyelitis was likely. This so-called "probe to bone" test was relatively specific (85%) and had a positive predictive value of 89% [5]. These results, as well as the simplicity of the test, make this procedure very useful in clinical practice, and it has been adopted widely. However, the pretest probability was high in the study population, and sensitivity was only 66%. Further evidence is needed to justify its use as the sole criterion in diagnosing osteomyelitis. Moreover, the low negative predictive value of these two physical examination findings certainly makes it difficult to exclude osteomyelitis using clinical evaluation alone.

Laboratory studies

Laboratory evaluation is of limited usefulness in diagnosing diabetic foot osteomyelitis. Leukocytosis is infrequent, occurring in fewer than 50% of those affected [21,25]. An elevated erythrocyte sedimentation rate or C-reactive protein is sensitive for bone infection, but the specificity of such a finding is questionable [4,26–28].

Imaging studies

A number of imaging modalities is reported to be useful for diagnosing osteomyelitis in the diabetic foot. Relatively inexpensive and easy to obtain, plain radiographs are the initial diagnostic study of choice. Characteristic findings of osteomyelitis include periosteal reaction followed by focal erosion of cortical or medullary bone. Unfortunately, these changes are generally not evident on plain films until 40% to 70% of the bone has been resorbed, reducing the sensitivity in the first 2 to 4 weeks of infection. In addition, these changes may be indistinguishable from those of neuropathic osteoarthropathy. These limitations reduce the sensitivity and specificity of plain radiographs to approximately 66% and 60%, respectively, according to a review by Lipsky [8]. Although not often useful in diagnosing osteomyelitis in the setting of acute infection, plain radiography becomes fairly specific and clinically useful when the initial results are normal, and subsequent films show characteristic changes over time. This is especially true if the involved area underlies an infected ulcer or if bone can be probed in the base of the wound. Also, plain x-rays may show gas in soft tissues, bony deformity, generalized Charcot changes, or fracture.

When plain films are negative, radionuclide bone scanning can be useful to evaluate the diabetic foot for osteomyelitis. Technetium-99 methylene diphosphonate scans can show abnormalities of bone turnover earlier than plain films can, resulting in an average sensitivity approaching 90% for three- or four-phase scans [8,29]. However, because turnover is increased in most bone disorders (neuropathic osteoarthropathy, healing infection), the specificity of this test is poor, averaging less than 50% [4,8,29]. Labeled white blood cells (usually indium-111–labeled leukocytes) accumulate in areas of infection rather than bone turnover. As a result, while retaining the sensitivity of technetium scans [8,29], labeled white blood cell scans have much better specificity for osteomyelitis (averaging approximately 80%) [8,29–31]. Furthermore, as infection resolves, the labeled leukocyte uptake decreases and then normalizes, making it useful for assessing response to therapy [4]. In addition to being expensive and time consuming, the primary technical limitation of labeled white blood cell studies is the lack of anatomic resolution. Performing a traditional bone scan along with the WBC scan may slightly improve specificity by allowing differentiation of osteomyelitis from soft-tissue infection alone [29]. Combination bone and leukocyte scans are also useful for differentiating osteomyelitis from neuropathic osteoarthropathy. Two recent studies reported very high specificity for detection of bone infection, despite the presence of concurrent neuropathic osteoarthropathy in the patient populations [30,31].

Magnetic resonance imaging (MRI) is the most widely used modality for investigating possible diabetic foot osteomyelitis. Sensitivity of MRI is very high, generally reported to be between 90% and 100%, whereas specificity ranges between 80% and 100% in most studies [8,28,32–34]. MRI diagnosis of osteomyelitis is based on altered bone marrow signal. Marrow infection results in loss of fat and its normally bright signal on T_1-weighted images, as well as edema, which increases signal intensity on T_2-weighted or STIR images. Unfortunately, although these changes are highly sensitive for osteomyelitis, a number of pathologic conditions such as fracture, tumor, inflammatory arthritis, neuropathic osteoarthropathy, or recent postoperative changes can result in similar bone marrow signal changes. To increase the specificity, MRI results then must be correlated with the overall clinical picture. When these classic changes occur in the absence of a fracture line or discrete lesion but in the vicinity of ulceration, sinus tract, or soft-tissue infection, the specificity for bone infection is increased [32–34].

Although expensive, MRI offers excellent anatomic detail and spatial resolution compared with other imaging modalities. This advantage allows it to demonstrate the extent of both bone and soft-tissue infection in the diabetic foot, knowledge that may be very useful for operative planning and foot salvage [33]. Osseous extent is best determined on T_1 images and can be overdiagnosed on T_2 or enhanced images [34].

Biopsy and bone culture

Bone biopsy and culture often are used as the gold standard for identification of diabetic osteomyelitis. Percutaneous samples can be harvested under fluoroscopic or computed tomography guidance using a core biopsy needle through uninvolved skin. This technique is considered safe and to have a high diagnostic accuracy [8,24,35,36]. The use of lidocaine to obtain specimens does not seem to interfere with results [37]. The second method for obtaining material for biopsy is surgical excision. Whenever bone is resected from the diabetic foot, it should undergo both histologic examination along with Gram stain and culture. Histologic evidence of osteomyelitis consists of acute or chronic inflammatory cells along with bone fragmentation and necrosis.

The advantage of biopsy is its potential to provide culture and antimicrobial susceptibility data. Bone cultures often do not correlate with soft-tissue samples, and bone biopsy has been shown to be more useful for guiding antibiotic therapy versus soft-tissue culture alone [38]. In spite of this advantage, the frequent clinical use of bone biopsy outside of the operating room is controversial. The procedure is expensive and invasive, and results may not be available for several days. In addition, small bones of the foot can yield poor core needle specimens and previous suppressive antibiotic therapy, and patchy bone involvement can lead to false-negative results. As a result, biopsy often is reserved for difficult cases or cases in which the causative organism and susceptibility are believed to be necessary to guide treatment.

Osteomyelitis versus neuropathic osteoarthropathy

Differentiation between osteomyelitis and neuro-osteoarthropathy (Charcot arthropathy) is a common diagnostic dilemma. The two conditions present with similar clinical and radiologic findings. Furthermore, because both typically owe their origin to peripheral neuropathy, the same patient population is at risk for both disorders, and both can be present in the same foot.

Although difficult, distinguishing the two disorders is important because they are treated very differently. Clinically, both osteomyelitis and Charcot arthropathy can present with swelling, warmth, and edema of the affected area. The dependent erythema of neuro-osteoarthropathy is said to improve with elevation, whereas that of cellulitis will not [39]. The presence or absence of skin breakdown is most helpful clinically in distinguishing these two conditions. Osteomyelitis is almost always preceded by a neuropathic skin ulcer and is most common in the forefoot. Neuropathic osteoarthropathy, however, is found much more commonly in the midfoot. Skin breakdown is rare and occurs typically as a complication of the later stages of the disease when deformity is present.

The plain film appearance of these two disorders has considerable overlap, and films may show negative results initially in both situations. Fragmentation, polyostotic involvement, and joint subluxation occur more commonly in Charcot disease, whereas osteomyelitis results in progressive destruction and periosteal reaction [40]. Differentiation of these conditions by MRI is better than with plain films but remains problematic. Osteomyelitis is more likely when changes are focal, centered within bone itself, and associated with adjacent ulcer, cellulitis, abscess, or sinus tract. Neuropathic osteoarthropathy is more likely with multiple foci or when changes are limited to joints, subchondral bone, and juxta-articular soft tissues [32]. In difficult cases, bone biopsy and culture or combined indium-labeled leukocyte/technetium bone scans may be necessary to arrive at a diagnosis.

Treating osteomyelitis

The management of osteomyelitis in the diabetic foot is complicated and controversial. Level one or two studies comparing management options are rare or nonexistent. Variations in patient populations and diagnostic criteria for osteomyelitis make analysis of retrospective case series difficult. As in most conditions, a spectrum of severity exists, and each infection occurs under different patient circumstances. Therefore, treatment must be individualized to each patient. For these reasons, clinician judgment as well as patient preferences are very important in selecting the best management plan.

Multidisciplinary management

Diabetes mellitus is a multisystem disease, and its treatment requires a multidisciplinary team approach [1]. Comprehensive medical treatment by the patient's primary care physician and medical specialists should be continued or instituted. Control of hyperglycemia is well known to be more difficult in the setting of an acute infection, but it must be optimized, because leukocyte dysfunction correlates with blood glucose levels [11,41]. Other systemic effects and comorbidities of diabetes should be assessed and addressed. Nephropathy, poor nutrition, and smoking can decrease immune function and delay wound healing and should be managed aggressively [21,42,43]. Basic diabetic foot care should be arranged including screening, patient education, footwear, and ongoing skin and nail care.

Vascular evaluation is critical to the management of the diabetic foot infection and has a major impact on outcome. Peripheral vascular occlusive disease is more common among patients with diabetes mellitus, can contribute to ulcer formation, and worsens the prognosis both for wound healing and limb salvage in patients with osteomyelitis of the foot [44]. Patients with absent or diminished pulses or those with other signs of vascular insufficiency, such as claudication, rest pain, skin changes, or poor capillary refill should undergo further evaluation, usually with arterial Doppler ultrasound or transcutaneous oxygen diffusion. Evidence of significant arterial compromise of the limb should prompt evaluation by a vascular surgeon. Diabetes alone does not portend a worse outcome for surgical revascularization [45,59]. In fact, for patients with osteomyelitis of the foot, aggressive arterial reconstruction has been shown to result in both improved wound healing and a fivefold increase in limb salvage [44].

Conservative therapy with antibiotics and limited debridement

Traditionally, osteomyelitis in the diabetic patient has mandated surgical resection followed by intravenous antibiotics. Infected, necrotic bone has been labeled a "foreign body" that must be excised to healthy bone to achieve healing. Early attempts at management with antibiotics alone yielded poor results [46]. A number of series have suggested better outcomes with early operative intervention. Karchmer and Gibbons [47], in a review of diabetic patients with histologically confirmed osteomyelitis, reported that early surgical resection of involved bone followed by short-term intravenous antibiotics achieved an 88% cure rate and preserved a weight-bearing surface in all patients. Tan et al. [48] found a decreased rate of above-ankle amputation and shorter hospital stay for patients receiving aggressive surgical intervention in the first 3 days of hospitalization versus antibiotic therapy alone. Henke and colleagues [44] found prolonged outpatient antibiotic use to be associated with decreased wound healing and limb salvage, whereas early surgical intervention improved healing more than intravenous antibiotics alone.

Recently, however, there has been growing interest in the treatment of diabetic osteomyelitis using antibiotics, either alone or in combination with limited local debridement [49]. Proponents of this method point to earlier diagnosis of bone infections using MRI, increased efficacy of newer antibiotics in penetrating bone and glycocalix biofilms, as well as poor results reported in some surgical case series. A number of published case series have attempted to evaluate the efficacy of conservative management for suspected or confirmed osteomyelitis. These series, encompassing more than 500 patients, have been reviewed by Jeffcoate and Lipsky [8,24]. The studies vary in their patient population, method of diagnosis, antibiotic regimen, definition of remission, and extent of local debridement, which makes generalization difficult. Reported remission rates vary from 25% to 88%, with the majority reporting satisfactory results and recommending this option in selected patients. Pittet and colleagues [50] treated 50 patients who had deep foot infection and suspected osteomyelitis using local ulcer debridement and prolonged antibiotic therapy. Thirty-five (70%) patients' infections healed completely with no sign of relapse during the 2-year follow-up. Prior hospitalization for foot lesions, signs of systemic infection, renal insufficiency, and gangrene predicted failure of conservative management [50]. Thus, as is the case in many foot and ankle disorders, a trial of nonoperative treatment for osteomyelitis of the diabetic foot may be a good option for many patients. The clinician must remember, however, that antibiotic treatment is not without complications, and surgical intervention is warranted in many cases. Prospective, randomized studies are needed to resolve this issue and to evaluate the relative efficacy of operative versus nonoperative treatment for given patient populations.

Regardless of whether surgery is performed, antibiotic therapy is essential to the management of diabetic osteomyelitis. Initial therapy is empiric. A number of agents, including clindamycin, imipenem/cilastatin, fluoroquinolones, cephalosporins, linezolid, and penicillin/β-lactamase inhibitor combinations have shown clinical effectiveness, but no single agent or combination has been proven to be most effective [51]. Any empiric regimen should cover staphylococci and streptococci. Recurrent, unresponsive, or severe cases may need gram-negative and Enterococcus coverage, whereas necrotic or foul-smelling wounds may warrant anti-anaerobic agents. If bone culture and sensitivity results become available, specific therapy should be initiated, including vancomycin for methicillin-resistant staphylococci.

Parenteral therapy for at least 6 weeks traditionally is recommended for diabetic osteomyelitis, although no good evidence exists to guide the duration of therapy or the timing of switching to an oral agent. Oral agents with good bioavailability such fluoroquinolones may be as effective as parenteral therapy [52]. If all infected bone is excised, treatment as a soft-tissue infection for 1 to 2 weeks may be acceptable [8,22,51].

Most infected ulcers should undergo sharp local debridement through their entire thickness, whether in an outpatient setting, at the bedside, or in the operating room. All devitalized tissue and debris should be removed, and pus should be drained. Undermined skin edges can create environments suitable for bacterial proliferation and should also be excised, allowing better assessment of underlying infection. Whenever possible, round wounds should be converted to more elliptical ones, which heal more readily.

Surgical treatment

The basic philosophy in the surgical treatment of diabetic foot infections should be foot salvage, that is, the preservation of the maximum amount of functional foot [39]. In the setting of deep infection in the diabetic foot, the temptation often exists to remove the problem by performing a "definitive" amputation. This approach certainly is indicated in some circumstances. However, a below-knee amputation is not necessarily definitive. Only about 60% of diabetic above-ankle amputees achieve ambulation with a prosthesis [53]. As a result of systemic involvement and excessive weight bearing on the uninvolved limb, up to 50% of patients with severe diabetic foot infections will acquire a similar infection in the contralateral foot, many of which will lead to a second amputation and further loss of mobility [54].

Despite the possibility of remission with antibiotics alone, a large number of diabetic patients with a deep foot infection will require surgical intervention. Severe infections pose a threat to the limb as well as to the patient's life. The presence of systemic signs or symptoms (eg, fever, tachycardia, hypotension, and vomiting) suggesting sepsis should prompt urgent surgical debridement. Abscesses of the foot must be drained. For this purpose, longitudinal incisions allow easier extension, and plantar incisions should be avoided, if possible. Patients with diabetic neuropathy can have higher foot compartment pressures than healthy individuals. Infection and resultant edema can lead to compartment syndrome, necessitating immediate surgical release to minimize necrosis [55]. Necrotizing fasciitis is a rapidly spreading, destructive, polymicrobial soft-tissue infection that has been associated with diabetes mellitus. Affected patients typically exhibit intense pain that is out of proportion to examination findings, high fever, tachycardia, leukocytosis, and skin blistering. Early diagnosis and emergent surgical debridement of all affected tissue are necessary to lessen the high mortality rate [56].

In the absence of sepsis or severe soft-tissue infection, a more conservative and elective approach can be considered for mild and moderate infections. Despite the option of conservative treatment, it may be determined that infected bone must be excised. Debridement is preferable to amputation, if possible. The metatarsal heads are the most frequent sites involved in diabetic foot osteomyelitis, and limited resection in this area may be possible. The preferred approach is through a separate surgical incision, not through the infected wound or ulcer itself, avoiding incisions on the plantar surface of the foot [39]. This second wound can then be closed loosely with nonabsorbable sutures. If deformity is believed to have contributed to ulceration and infection (eg, varus deformity or Achilles contracture), the underlying deformity must be corrected by bracing or surgical treatment for healing to occur. Metatarsal head resection can lead to transfer lesions, but this risk can be reduced by appropriate footwear and insoles and should not preclude the trial of this more conservative option. After debridement, meticulous wound care and wound offloading, with consideration of total contact casting, should be instituted to promote healing.

Despite advancements in care of the diabetic foot, amputation is still necessary in many cases. Rather than a treatment failure, amputation should be viewed as an opportunity for limb salvage with the goal of producing a functional, energy-efficient lower extremity. Before amputation, vascular status should be evaluated for both the likelihood of healing at the planned amputation site and the possibility of a more distal amputation with revascularization. A balance must be achieved between resecting sufficient bone and soft tissue to cure infection and allow closure while preserving stability of the residual foot. Leaving large wounds to heal by secondary intention is debilitating for the patient. Second-look operations and revision amputations may be necessary.

A more limb-conserving amputation is almost always desirable. The amputation level is related directly to efficiency of ambulation. Energy is at a premium in the diabetic population because of frequency of heart disease and other comorbidities. Conservation of even the proximal phalanx reduces drift of the other toes and preserves at least partial function of the plantar fascia, especially in the hallux. Medial or lateral ray resections typically require less bracing than transmetatarsal amputations. When the forefoot is not salvageable by local amputation, transtarsal amputation or Syme ankle disarticulation are desirable alternatives. These options preserve efficiency of ambulation, functional independence, and possibly lifespan more consistently than below-knee amputation. Both procedures have been shown recently to achieve successful healing in diabetic patients with infection or gangrene, as long as vascular and nutritional criteria for good wound healing are met [57,58]. Local muscle flaps and microvascular free flaps have also been shown to be helpful adjuncts for foot salvage after diabetic foot infection, because outcome does not appear to be adversely affected by diabetes [58,59].

Despite the desirability of foot salvage, prosthetic replacement may be preferable to a poorly functioning foot, particularly if it improves mobility.

Although the quality of life of a diabetic amputee is lower than diabetic controls, it is usually better than that of the patient with a chronic foot ulcer, especially a chronically infected ulcer [57]. Thus, attempts at conservative treatment should not extend indefinitely, and below-knee amputation may be the best or only alternative for some patients. Clearly, regardless of the treatment options under consideration, the patient must be involved heavily in the decision process and should have a good understanding of the risks and benefits of each alternative.

Summary

Neuropathic ulceration and altered immune function place the diabetic patient at increased risk for polymicrobial osteomyelitis of the foot and ankle. The optimal method for evaluation and management of this difficult condition is controversial, and further studies are needed. Infected ulcers with exposed or palpable bone can be assumed to have underlying osteomyelitis. Although plain films should be ordered in each case, MRI is most often used for evaluation and surgical planning. Difficult cases, such as those associated with Charcot osteoarthropathy, may require labeled leukocyte scanning or bone biopsy to arrive at the diagnosis. A multidisciplinary team approach is best, allowing optimal treatment of all associated conditions that commonly affect patients with diabetes mellitus. Vascular evaluation and intervention are critical in the presence of vascular insufficiency or ischemia. Empiric, usually broad-spectrum antibiotics and meticulous local wound care may achieve remission of mild-to-moderately severe infections and should be included in all treatment regimens. Severe infection, ischemia, or sepsis requires an aggressive surgical approach. Bone resection, correction of deformity, or amputation often are necessary and should be done with the goal of salvaging a functional foot.

References

[1] Pinzur MS, Slovenkai MP, Trepman E, et al. Diabetes Committee of American Orthopaedic Foot and Ankle Society. Guidelines for diabetic foot care: recommendations endorsed by the Diabetes Committee of the American Orthopaedic Foot and Ankle Society. Foot Ankle Int 2005;26(1):113–9.

[2] Pecoraro RE, Reiber G, Burgess EM. Pathways to diabetic limb amputation; basis for prevention. Diabetes Care 1990;13(5):513–21.

[3] Tennvall GR, Apelqvist J. Health economic consequences of diabetic foot lesions. Clin Infect Dis 2004;39(S2):S132–9.

[4] Newman LG, Waller J, Palestro CJ, et al. Unsuspected osteomyelitis in diabetic foot ulcers. Diagnosis and monitoring by leukocyte scanning with indium in 111 oxyquinoline. JAMA 1991;266(9):1246–51.

[5] Grayson ML, Gibbons GW, Balogh K, et al. Probing to bone in infected pedal ulcers. A clinical sign of underlying osteomyelitis in diabetic patients. JAMA 1995;273(9):721–3.

[6] Calhoun JH, Mader JT. Osteomyelitis of the diabetic foot. In: Frykberg RG, editor. The high risk foot in diabetes mellitus. New York: Churchill Livingstone; 1991. p. 213–40.

[7] Boyko EJ, Ahroni JH, Stensel V, et al. A prospective study of risk factors for diabetic foot ulcer. Diabetes Care 1999;229(7):1036–42.

[8] Lipsky BA. Osteomyelitis of the foot in diabetic patients. Clin Infect Dis 1997;25(6): 1318–26.

[9] Reiber GE, Vileikyte L, Boyko EJ, et al. Causal pathways for incident lower-extremity ulcers in patients with diabetes. Diabetes Care 1999;22(1):157–62.

[10] Shah BR, Hux JE. Quantifying the risk of infectious diseases for people with diabetes-Diabetes Care 2003;26(2):510–3.

[11] Delmaire M, Maugendre D, Moreno M, et al. Impaired leukocyte function in diabetic patients. Diabet Med 1997;14(1):29–34.

[12] Kuusela P. Fibronectin binds to Staphylococcus aureus. Nature 1978;276(5689):718–20.

[13] Ciampolini J, Harding KG. Pathophysiology of chronic bacterial osteomyelitis. Why do antibiotics fail so often? Postgrad Med J 2000;76(898):479–83.

[14] Lerner UH, Sundqvist G, Ohlin A, et al. Bacteria inhibit biosynthesis of bone matrix proteins in human osteoblasts. Clin Orthop 1998;346:244–54.

[15] Ge Y, MacDonald H, Lipsky B, et al. Microbiological profile of infected diabetic foot ulcers. Diabet Med 2002;19(12):1032–4.

[16] Lavery LA, Sariaya M. Microbiology of osteomyelitis in diabetic foot ulcers. J Foot Ankle Surg 1995;34(1):61–4.

[17] Senneville E, Hugues M, Beltrand E, et al. Culture of percutaneous bone biopsy specimens for diagnosis of diabetic foot osteomyelitis: concordance with ulcer swab cultures. Clin Infect Dis 2006;42(1):57–62.

[18] Dang CN, Prasad YDM, Boulton AJM, et al. Methicillin-resistant Staphylococcus aureus in the diabetic foot clinic: a worsening problem. Diabet Med 2003;20(2):159–61.

[19] Game FL, Boswell T, Soar C, et al. MRSA Outcome in diabetic foot ulcers with and without MRSA. Diabet Med 2003;20(S2):30.

[20] Hartemann-Heurtier A, Robert J, Jacqueminet S, et al. Diabetic foot ulcer and multidrug-resistant organisms: risk factors and impact. Diabet Med 2004;21(7):710–5.

[21] Eneroth M, Apelqvist J, Stenstrom A. Clinical characteristics and outcome in 223 diabetic patients with deep foot infections. Foot Ankle Int 1997;18(11):716–22.

[22] Frykberg RG. An evidence based approach to diabetic foot infections. Am J Surg 2003; 186(5A):44S–54S.

[23] Wagner FW Jr. The diabetic foot. Orthopedics 1987;10(1):163–72.

[24] Jeffcoate WJ, Lipsky BA. Controversies in diagnosing and managing osteomyelitis of the foot in diabetes. Clin Infect Dis 2004;39(S2):S115–22.

[25] Armstrong DG, Lavery LA, Sariaya M, et al. Leukocytosis is a poor indicator of acute osteomyelitis of the foot in diabetes mellitus. J Foot Ankle Surg 1996;35(4):280–3.

[26] Jacobson AF, Harley JD, Lipsky BA, et al. Diagnosis of osteomyelitis in the presence of soft-tissue infection and radiologic evidence of osseous abnormalities: value of leukocyte scintigraphy. AJR Am J Roentgenol 1991;57(4):807–12.

[27] Eneroth M, Larsson J, Apelqvist J. Deep foot infections in patients with diabetes and foot ulcer: an entity with different characteristics, treatments, and prognosis. J Diabetes Complicat 1999;13(5–6):254–63.

[28] Eckman MH, Greenfield S, Mackey WC, et al. Foot infections in diabetic patients. Decision and cost-effectiveness analyses. JAMA 1995;273(9):712–20.

[29] Johnson JE, Kennedy EJ, Shereff MJ, et al. Prospective study of bone, indium-111-labeled white blood cell, and gallium-67 scanning for the evaluation of osteomyelitis in the diabetic foot. Foot Ankle Int 1996;17(1):10–6.

[30] Unal SN, Birinci H, Baktiroglu S, et al. Comparison of Tc-99m methylene diphosphonate, Tc-99m human immune globulin, and Tc-99m-labeled white blood cell scintigraphy in the diabetic foot. Clin Nucl Med 2001;26(12):1016–21.

[31] Lipman BT, Collier BD, Carrera GF, et al. Detection of osteomyelitis in the neuropathic foot: nuclear medicine, MRI and conventional radiography. Clin Nucl Med 1998;23(2):77–82.

[32] Ledermann HP, Morrison WB. Differential diagnosis of pedal osteomyelitis and diabetic neuroarthropathy: MR imaging. Semin Musculoskelet Radiol 2005;9(3):272–83.

[33] Morrison WB, Schweitzer ME, Wapner KL, et al. Osteomyelitis in feet of diabetics: clinical accuracy, surgical utility, and cost-effectiveness of MR imaging. Radiology 1995;196(2): 557–64.

[34] Chatha DS, Cunningham PM, Schweitzer ME. MR imaging of the diabetic foot: diagnostic challenges. Radiol Clin North Am 2005;43(4):747–59.

[35] Howard CB, Einhorn M, Dagan R, et al. Fine-needle bone biopsy to diagnose osteomyelitis. J Bone Joint Surg Br 1994;76(2):311–4.

[36] Mushlin AI, Littenberg B. Diagnosing pedal osteomyelitis: testing choices and their consequences. J Gen Intern Med 1994;9(1):1–7.

[37] Schweitzer ME, Deely DM, Beavis K, et al. Does the use of lidocaine affect the culture of percutaneous bone biopsy specimens obtained to diagnose osteomyelitis? An in vitro and in vivo study. AJR Am J Roentgenol 1995;164(5):1201–3.

[38] Khatri G, Wagner DK, Sohnle PG. Effect of bone biopsy in guiding antimicrobial therapy for osteomyelitis complicating open wounds. Am J Med Sci 2001;321(6):367–71.

[39] Brodsky JW. The diabetic foot. In: Mann RA, Coughlin MJ, editors. Surgery of the foot and ankle. 7th edition (volume 2). St. Louis (MO): Mosby; 1999. p. 877–958.

[40] Berendt AR, Lipsky B. Is this bone infected or not? Differentiating neuro-osteoarthropathy from osteomyelitis in the diabetic foot. Curr Diab Rep 2004;4(6):424–9.

[41] Osar Z, Samanci T, Demirel GY, et al. Nicotinamide effects oxidative burst activity of neutrophils in patients with poorly controlled type 2 diabetes mellitus. Exp Diabesity Res 2004;5(2):155–62.

[42] Griffiths GD, Wieman TJ. The influence of renal function on diabetic foot ulceration. Arch Surg 1990;125(12):1567–9.

[43] Sorensen LT, Karlsmark T, Gottrup F. Abstinence from smoking reduces incisional wound infection: a randomized controlled trial. Ann Surg 2003;238(1):1–5.

[44] Henke PK, Blackburn SA, Wainess RW, et al. Osteomyelitis of the foot and toe in adults is a surgical disease: conservative management worsens lower extremity salvage. Ann Surg 2005;241(6):885–94.

[45] Pomposelli FB, Kansal N, Hamdan AD, et al. A decade of experience with dorsalis pedis artery bypass: analysis of outcome in more than 1000 cases. J Vasc Surg 2003;37(2):307–15.

[46] Waldvogel FA, Papageorgiou PS. Osteomyelitis: the past decade. N Engl J Med 1980 14;303(7)360–70.

[47] Karchmer AW, Gibbons GW. Foot infections in diabetes: evaluation and management. Curr Clin Top Infect Dis 1994;14:1–22.

[48] Tan JS, Friedman NM, Hazelton-Miller C, et al. Can aggressive treatment of diabetic foot infections reduce the need for above-ankle amputation? Clin Infect Dis 1999;23(2):286–91.

[49] American Diabetes Association. Consensus Development Conference on Diabetic Foot Wound Care: Boston, Massachusetts, April 7–8, 1999. Diabetes Care 1999;22(8):1354–60.

[50] Pittet D, Wyssa B, Herter-Clavel C, et al. Outcome of diabetic foot infections treated conservatively: a retrospective cohort study with long-term follow-up. Arch Intern Med 1999 26;159(8)851–6.

[51] Lipsky BA. Medical treatment of diabetic foot infections. Clin Infect Dis 2004;39(S2): S101–14.

[52] Kuck EM, Bouter KP, Hoekstra JB, et al. Tissue concentrations after a single-dose, orally administered ofloxacin in patients with diabetic foot infections. Foot Ankle Int 1998; 19(1):38–40.

[53] Van Damme H, Rorive M, Martens De Noorthout BM, et al. Amputations in diabetic patients: a plea for footsparing surgery. Acta Chir Belg 2001;101(3):123–9.

[54] Kucan JO, Robson MC. Diabetic foot infections: fate of the contralateral foot. Plast Reconstr Surg 1986;77(3):439–41.

[55] Maharaj D, Bahadursingh S, Shah D, et al. Sepsis and the scalpel: anatomic compartments and the diabetic foot. Vasc Endovascular Surg 2005;39(5):421–3.
[56] Childers BJ, Potyondy LD, Nachreiner R, et al. Necrotizing fasciitis: a fourteen-year retrospective study of 163 consecutive patients. Am Surg 2002;68(2):109–16.
[57] Price P. The diabetic foot: quality of life. Clin Infect Dis 2004;39:S129–31.
[58] Attinger CE, Ducic I, Cooper P, et al. The role of intrinsic muscle flaps of the foot for bone coverage in foot and ankle defects in diabetic and nondiabetic patients. Plast Reconstr Surg 2002;110(4):1047–54.
[59] Verhelle NA, Lemaire V, Nelissen X, et al. Combined reconstruction of the diabetic foot including revascularization and free-tissue transfer. J Reconstr Microsurg 2004;20(7):511–7.

ELSEVIER
SAUNDERS

Foot Ankle Clin N Am
11 (2006) 791–804

FOOT AND
ANKLE CLINICS

Lower-Extremity Amputations in Association with Diabetes Mellitus

Terrence M. Philbin, DO[a,b,c,*],
Gregory C. Berlet, MD[a,b], Thomas H. Lee, MD[a,b]

[a]Orthopedic Foot and Ankle Center, 6200 Cleveland Avenue, Suite 100, Columbus,
OH 43231, USA
[b]The Ohio State University College of Medicine and Public Health, 410 West 10th Avenue,
Columbus, OH 43210, USA
[c]Foot and Ankle Surgery, Grant Medical Center, 111 S. Grant Street, Columbus,
OH 43215, USA

The American Diabetes Association estimates that there are 20.8 million individuals, or 7% of the population, with diabetes mellitus in the United States; the condition is undiagnosed in approximately 6.2 million of these individuals [1]. In 2002, 224,092 deaths were related to diabetes, and that year the estimated cost of diabetes was $132 billion, or one of every 10 health care dollars spent in the United States [1].

Approximately 82,000 amputations related to diabetes mellitus were performed in 2002. Greater than 60% of all lower-extremity amputations are performed in diabetic patients, and the incidence of amputation among diabetic patients is 10 times that of the nondiabetic population [1]. Men with diabetes are 1.4 to 2.7 times more likely to require an amputation than are women with diabetes, and the likelihood of a lower-extremity amputation is increased 1.8-fold among Mexican Americans, 2.7-fold for African Americans, and 3-fold for Native Americans over whites [1]. In addition, morbid obesity has been correlated strongly with diabetes-associated foot morbidity [2].

In the past, amputations were considered a failure of treatment and the commencement of a life with disability and disfigurement. Fortunately, these views have changed, and patients now can accept amputation as a means of getting on with their lives. For the diabetic patient, an amputation can mark the beginning of a comprehensive rehabilitation process.

---

* Corresponding author. Orthopedic Foot and Ankle Center, 6200 Cleveland Avenue, Suite 100, Columbus, OH 43231.

E-mail address: philbsgoirish@wowway.com (T.M. Philbin).

1083-7515/06/$ - see front matter © 2006 Elsevier Inc. All rights reserved.
doi:10.1016/j.fcl.2006.06.012

foot.theclinics.com

Advancements in diagnosis, surgical techniques, postoperative rehabilitation, and orthotic and prosthetic devices have improved the outcomes for diabetic amputees over the years.

Nonetheless, it is well known that 30% of amputees lose their contralateral limb within 3 years and, after the amputation of a leg, approximately two thirds of patients die within 5 years [3]. Only 50% of patients who have a major amputation use a prosthesis [4].

Patient education about diabetes mellitus remains paramount in the prevention of amputations. Smith and colleagues [5] recently showed that minor environmental trauma can play a big role in diabetic amputation rates, and its avoidance should be emphasized in diabetic education. Wachtel [6] showed that poverty accounted for the differences in lower-extremity diabetic amputation rates of minorities 50 years old or older.

The main goal of amputation surgery is to salvage the greatest amount of functional limb that will heal. The energy expended when walking with a residual limb is inversely proportional to the length of the remaining limb and number of preserved joints. Patients with partial foot amputations require less energy to walk than patients with transtibial amputations. Smith [7] pointed out that occasionally the most distal amputation is not the wisest choice. For example, a nonambulatory patient with a knee flexion contracture may enjoy more successful outcome from a more proximal amputation at or above the knee than a below-knee amputation.

The amputee must have the cognitive abilities to understand and actively participate in the rehabilitation process. Patients must possess the hand strength and coordination to attach and remove a prosthetic device. In many cases, patients with partial foot amputations can wear near-normal shoes, preserving near-normal functions. Proper orthotic and prosthetic devices for partial foot amputations have been described previously [3].

Surgical decision making for the amputation level

One of the key decisions necessary for a successful outcome after diabetic amputation surgery is determining the level that will heal and become functional. The preoperative evaluation should include a clinical examination assessing the quality of the tissue; the extent of infection; amount of vascularity; and the patient's nutritional, immune, and ambulatory statuses [8]. Although no test for assessing the perfusion status of a lower extremity is 100% accurate, the currently accepted parameters indicating good healing potential for diabetic patients after an amputation are an ankle-brachial index of 0.5 or a transcutaneous partial pressure of oxygen ($TcPo_2$) between 20 and 30 mm Hg (edema, cellulitis, and the changes of venous outflow abnormalities can hamper the $TcPo_2$ reading) [2,7–9]. If the blood flow in the involved extremity is deemed poor, a vascular consult may be necessary. Ohsawa and coauthors [10] found skin thermography to be an important tool in deciding the level of an amputation and in avoiding reamputation.

From a nutritional standpoint, the currently accepted wound-healing parameter is a serum albumin level of 3.0 g/dL. A total lymphocyte count of greater than 1500 indicates immunocompetence for wound healing. Pinzur and coworkers [9] found 88% overall healing rate in 83 diabetic patients after Syme amputations and a serum albumin threshold of 2.5g/dL. For elderly patients in particular, avoiding multiple surgeries is important; thus, the initial surgery level should be planned with care. Amputation levels are shown in Fig. 1.

Lower-extremity amputation levels

Toe amputations

Amputations of the greater hallux and the lesser toes are the most common partial foot amputations. Diabetes mellitus is the most common etiology resulting in a toe amputation, accounting for approximately 24% of all diabetic amputations [11,12]. The skin incisions for toe amputations can be either side-to-side or plantar-to-dorsal, which allows the surgeon to use the best soft tissue available (Fig. 2). Typically, enough bone should be removed to allow for a tension-free closure. When performing a great toe amputation, it is important to preserve as much length as possible. If a great toe

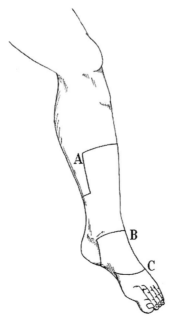

Fig. 1. Surgical levels for transtibial (*A*), Syme (*B*), and transmetatarsal (*C*) amputations. (Courtesy of Peter Maurus, MD, Columbus, Ohio.)

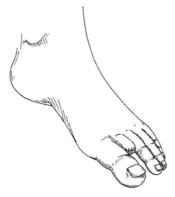

Fig. 2. Toe amputation performed with a side-to-side incision. (Courtesy of Peter Maurus, MD, Columbus, Ohio.)

amputation leaves a minimum length of 1 cm at the base of the proximal phalanx, the insertions of the plantar fascia, sesamoids, and flexor hallucis brevis remain intact. This enables some of the weight bearing of the first ray to be preserved, reducing extra pressure that could be transferred to the neighboring metatarsal heads [13]. After amputation of the greater hallux, pressures under the first metatarsal, lesser metatarsal heads, and remaining toes increases the risk of reulceration and further amputation [14]. When amputating the lesser toes, saving the base of the proximal phalanx may help to prevent migration of the neighboring toes. Second toe amputations should be done with caution because of the possible occurrence of a hallux valgus deformity [15].

Nehler and colleagues [16] reviewed the intermediate-term results of primary digit amputations in 92 diabetic patients with forefoot sepsis and adequate circulatory status. The primary healing rate was only 39%; infection remained in 76% of the patients, and an average of 1.0 reoperations and 1.6 hospitalizations were needed to treat those with a failed outcome. The investigators concluded that more extensive bony and soft tissue imaging, delayed or partial amputation closure at the time of the initial surgery, and a team approach, including infectious disease consult, would help increase the success rate.

Ray amputations

A ray resection includes a toe amputation and all or a portion of a metatarsal. In most cases, ray amputations are more durable and functional than a transmetatarsal amputation. As a general rule, no more than two rays should be resected to help preserve forefoot stability [15]. Multiple ray resections can cause substantial narrowing of the forefoot, which can make postoperative shoe wear difficult. The bases of the metatarsals should be preserved to prevent instability to the Lisfranc joint [15]. Unfortunately, in the diabetic population it is not always possible to adhere to these guidelines. In general, partial lateral foot amputations are well tolerated compared with partial medial amputations. Amputations of the first ray tend to increase load to the adjacent rays. Loss of the anterior tibialis insertion from the first ray may weaken ankle dorsiflexion and cause pronation of the foot. Fifth ray amputations are the most common and can be the most successful as well. Often, infected ulcers will form on the plantar and lateral aspects of the fifth metatarsal head. Smith [7] describes a racquet-shaped incision that allows the fifth toe, ulcer, and infected fifth metatarsal to be removed near the base. In the event the entire fifth metatarsal needs to be resected, the peroneal brevis should be reattached to allow for eversion.

Transmetatarsal amputation

Transmetatarsal amputations (TMA) are performed approximately 10,000 times annually in the United States (Fig. 3) [17]. In 1949 McKittrick and coauthors [18] first reported TMA as an alternative to transtibial amputation. Transmetatarsal amputation is associated with a decreased mortality rate when compared with higher-level amputations. Transmetatarsal amputation is preferred over transtibial amputation because TMA requires less energy for ambulation and it allows patients to have a distal weight-bearing residuum [19]. Sanders and Dunlap [19] reported an 83.3% success rate based on well-healed residual functional limbs. Cohen and colleagues [20] reported a 93.3% successful outcome in their TMA population, whereas Geroulakos and May [21] reported a 68% success rate. These investigators all agree that proper patient selection, heel cord lengthening, tendon

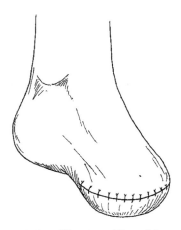

Fig. 3. Transmetatarsal amputation. (Courtesy of Peter Maurus, MD, Columbus, Ohio.)

transfers when necessary, and a suitable plantar flap, help prevent the pitfalls of TMA. Smith [7] described the importance of assessing muscle balance preoperatively to decide if Achilles tendon lengthening and/or tendon transfer would be required. Thomas and coauthors [22] reported retrospectively that their nondiabetic TMA patients' wounds healed significantly better compared with the diabetic patients' wounds.

Surgical failure of TMA is defined as a nonhealing wound or the need of a reamputation more proximally within 3 months of the primary procedure. Several studies report failure rates of TMA between 7% and 76% [20,23–26]. Sage and coworkers [26] reported 28% of 64 patients had early wound problems within 3 weeks of the procedure, and 14% had ulcerations during the year after surgery. Miller and colleagues [25] reported 27% of 107 TMA patients had wound complications and 28% needed a more proximal amputation. In the majority of these studies, diabetic neuropathy was the most common reason for having wound complications. In a prospective study, Eneroth and coworkers [27] found that 90% of their transtibial amputees were malnourished. Supplementary nutrition was found to improve wound healing in transtibial amputation patients, but the mortality rate was not affected.

Proper technique for a TMA should follow several guidelines. It is usually best to have a longer plantar flap, but in some cases flaps may be equal depending on the soft tissue defects. Normally, the dorsal incision is made 1 cm distal to the intended bony cut. Full-thickness flaps from skin down to bone are helpful for long-term healing. The flaps should be contoured from medial-distal to lateral-proximal so that the lateral side is shorter corresponding to the level of bony resection. The bony resections should be cut to recreate proper cascade effect. The blade should cut the bone from dorsal-distal to plantar-proximal to help prevent any pressure affect on an insensate foot. Early [4] describes the importance of making the bony cut 3 cm from the second metatarsal base in more proximal TMAs in an effort to maintain stability at the Lisfranc joint. A no-touch closure technique should be used. Achilles tendon lengthening is almost always warranted. Postoperative casting, with 5° of dorsiflexion, will help control swelling and protect the residual limb.

Lisfranc amputations

French surgeon Jacques Lisfranc first described an amputation to treat forefoot gangrene [28]. He developed a reputation for his ability to perform the amputation in less than 1 minute. Today, the tarsometatarsal joint bears his name. The biomechanical elements of a Lisfranc amputation are a shorter anatomic lever arm than a TMA and a higher rate of equinovarus contracture. The problem with this malposition after a Lisfranc amputation is related to the unopposed inversion of the posterior tibialis if the peroneal brevis has been sacrificed.

The primary indication for a Lisfranc amputation is substantial soft tissue loss of the forefoot in which a TMA would not be successful. Early [4] describes excising through the joints of the first, third, fourth, and fifth metatarsal joints. He recommends keeping the second metatarsal base in place to preserve the stability of the medial cuneiform and the vast plantar ligaments. The fifth metatarsal base should be shelled out subperiosteally in an effort to help preserve the attachments of the peroneal brevis, peroneus tertius, and the plantar fascia. The preserved periosteal insertion can be advanced to the cuboid to help maintain eversion control of the foot. If encountered with the removal of the first metatarsal base, the peroneal longus and anterior tibialis can be sutured to the neighboring soft tissues. Achilles tendon lengthening is equally as important to consider in Lisfranc amputations.

Chopart amputation

Amputation at the level of the transverse tarsal joints, Chopart amputation, can be a good choice for diabetic patients who are minimal ambulators. The Chopart amputee has a shortened anatomic lever arm, decreased push-off, and difficulty with stability. Much like the Lisfranc amputation, equinovarus deformity can be a problem. Chopart amputation does offer the advantage of retaining the tibiotalar joint and a functional residual limb when compared with a more proximal amputation. Early [4] emphasized the need to maximize the plantar flap to accommodate for the usual problem with the length of the dorsal flap. Proper bony debulking should be done to prevent any residual bony prominences that can cause increased pressure postoperatively. Any attachment of the posterior tibial tendon should be released to help prevent a varus deformity. If possible, a tendon sling around the talar neck with the anterior tibial tendon medially and the extensor tendons laterally will help combat deformity. As with the other midfoot amputations, tendo Achilles lengthening is necessary.

Syme amputation

In 1843, Syme first described an amputation about the ankle joint [29] (Figs. 4 and 5). He stated that the number of limbs he removed could have been prevented with this operation as an alternative. Wagner [30] modified the original technique by performing it in two stages. Studies have found that a Syme amputation enables the patient to expend less energy during ambulation than those with more proximal limb amputations. A clear advantage of a Syme amputation is the potential of achieving a full load-bearing residual limb that is near normal in length. Current research has found the patients with a Syme amputation have less short-term morbidity and tend to live longer than patients with a higher-level amputation. In a multicenter review, Pinzur and coworkers [31] found the mortality rate

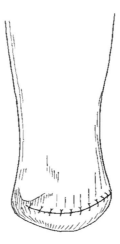

Fig. 4. Syme amputation. (Courtesy of Peter Maurus, MD, Columbus, Ohio.)

of Syme amputation patients to be approximately 33% at 5 years after surgery compared with a 33% death rate of transtibial amputation patients at 2 years postoperatively. Wagner [30] believed patients were candidates for a Syme amputation if they met certain criteria: good potential to ambulate with a prosthesis after surgery, a viable heel pad, no infection at the heel pad level, and adequate vascularity.

Wagner [30] modified Syme's original technique by doing the procedure in two stages. Stage one was an ankle disarticulation. Wagner believed that the distal tibial and fibula cartilage provided protection against infection and that leaving the cartilage intact prevented the heel pad from scarring into the distal tibia. Approximately 6 weeks after the wounds from stage one healed, Wagner would return to excise the malleoli in line with

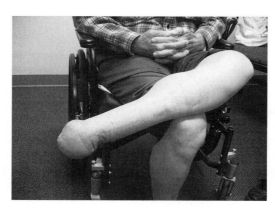

Fig. 5. Syme amputation.

the tibiotalar joint. He reported a 90% success rate, with 71% of the patients in his study returning to their presurgical functional levels. Pinzur and coauthors [32] compared the results of one-stage versus two-stage Syme amputation in patients with diabetic foot infections and found similar results. These investigators concluded that the two-stage procedure resulted in higher risk of perioperative medical complications owing to a second procedure and increased medical costs overall. In 2003, Pinzur and colleagues [9] reviewed retrospectively their results of 97 adult patients with diabetes mellitus who underwent a one-stage Syme amputation and found that the wounds healed in 84.5% of the patients. The infection rate was 23% and was three times greater among patients who were smokers. The majority of these infections were superficial and eventually healed with local wound care and antibiosis.

Heel-pad migration has been a problem reported in the literature. Pinzur and coworkers [9] recommend anchoring the heel pad to the distal tibia to prevent heel pad migration. Bollinger and Thordarson [33] reported good results in patients with large heel ulcers as an alternative to transtibial amputation and in patients who were not candidates for a Syme amputation.

Pinzur [34] has found that after a Syme amputation, patients have excellent proprioception when using a prosthesis with the residual limb, require little gait training, and that the residual limb rarely develops pain or ulceration.

Transtibial amputations

The transtibial amputation is the most common surgical amputation performed in the United States (Fig. 6). Fig. 7 shows an infected diabetic ulcer with osteomyelitis of the calcaneus that required a guillotine amputation (Fig. 8). The total cost of a transtibial amputation including hospitalization,

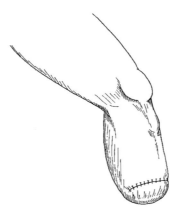

Fig. 6. Transtibial amputation. (Courtesy of Peter Maurus, MD, Columbus, Ohio.)

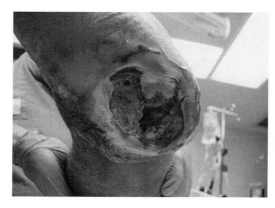

Fig. 7. Infected diabetic ulcer with osteomyelitis of the calcaneus required a guillotine amputation.

surgery, rehabilitation, physical therapy, and prosthetics often can exceed $50,000 [35]. Traditionally, surgeons and patients have viewed a transtibial amputation as a failure. Often, however, transtibial amputation can be successful and result in a patient's functional independence (Fig. 9).

In most cases, transtibial amputation can be accomplished by applying well-known principles and well-established surgical techniques. Consequently, and sometimes unfortunately, transtibial amputation often is the first case assigned to many junior residents. White and coauthors [36] retrospectively reviewed 193 lower limb amputations and found that patients were more likely to walk with a prosthesis if the amputation surgery was performed by a senior trainee compared with a junior trainee. Surgeons must follow appropriate guidelines for a successful outcome. A well-performed transtibial amputation can result in a high level of patient

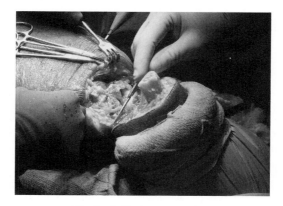

Fig. 8. Guillotine amputation.

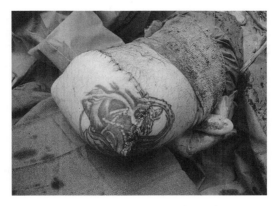

Fig. 9. Transtibial amputation preserving patient's tattoo.

satisfaction and function. The long posterior flap technique has become the most common based on its good success record. Other techniques have been described, including anteroposterior, sagittal, and skewed flaps. The level of the tibial cut should be as distal as possible down to the middle and distal third of the tibia. Distal-third amputations should be avoided because of the lack of adequate soft tissue coverage and the difficulty of prosthetic fitting. In the past, textbooks described the transtibial cut as being 15 cm from the knee joint. Today, as long as the tibial cut is above the distal third of the tibia, the surgeon should obtain as much length as the soft tissues dictate.

Smith [7] defined the goal of transtibial amputation as a cylindrically shaped residuum with muscle stabilization, distal tibial padding, and a nonpainful and nonadherent scar. The length of the posterior flap should equal the diameter of the soft tissue at the level of the tibial cut plus 1 cm. The fibula should be transected 1 to 2 cm proximal to the transtibial cut. Surgeons should assure that no bony spikes remain after the osseous cuts. All of the nerves should be transected with tension to allow retraction and to prevent painful neuromas. Myodesis of the posterior fascia to the anterior tibial periosteum can help combat retraction.

Postamputation care

Matsen and colleagues [37] retrospectively reviewed 148 patients with lower extremity amputation using questionnaires to determine the patients' perceptions of the outcome of the amputation. Patient satisfaction correlated with a comfortable residual limb, the condition of the contralateral limb, appearance and function of the prosthesis, and the ability to exercise. Younger patients and patients who could ambulate longer distances were more satisfied.

Larsson and coworkers [38] prospectively studied 189 diabetic patients who had either a minor amputation or a major amputation. The goal of the study was to evaluate the long-term outcome after minor and major amputation regarding survival, new amputation, and rehabilitation. The primary amputation level was considered minor if below the ankle and major if above the ankle. No Symes amputations were performed. The mean healing time was 29 weeks for the minor amputations and 8 weeks for the major amputations. The mortality rates at 1, 3, and 5 years after the primary amputation were 15%, 38%, and 68%, respectively. The rate of mortality was higher in the major amputation group that healed than in the minor amputation group that healed. The rate of new amputations after major and minor primary amputations was equal. The rehabilitation potential was lower for the major amputation group than the minor amputation.

Summary

Aksoy and coworkers [39] found that a multidisciplinary diabetic foot care team can help decrease the rate of major amputations and improve the patients' quality of life. Multidisciplinary care also includes proper patient education, which can help patients with diabetes mellitus control factors that can lead to complications, such as high blood glucose, high blood pressure, and increased lipid levels. The American Diabetes Association reports that such comprehensive foot care programs can reduce lower-extremity amputation rates among diabetic patients as much as 45% to 60% [1].

Acknowledgments

The authors acknowledge Janet L. Tremaine, ELS, Tremaine Medical Communications, for editorial assistance and thank Peter Maurus, MD, for creating the illustrations.

References

[1] American Diabetes Association. Diabetes statistics. Available at: www.diabetes.org/diabetes-statistics.jsp. Accessed December 28, 2005.
[2] Pinzur M, Freeland R, Juknelis D. The association between body mass index and foot disorders in diabetic patients. Foot Ankle Int 2005;26(5):375–7.
[3] Philbin TM, Leyes M, Sferra JJ, et al. Orthotic and prosthetic devices in partial foot amputations. Foot Ankle Clin 2001;6(2):215–28.
[4] Early JS. Transmetatarsal and midfoot amputations. Clin Orthop 1999;361:85–90.
[5] Smith DG, Assai M, Reiber GE, et al. Minor environmental trauma and lower extremity amputation in high-risk patients with diabetes: incidence, pivotal events, etiology, and amputation level in a prospectively followed cohort. Foot Ankle Int 2003;24(9):690–5.
[6] Wachtel MS. Family poverty accounts for differences in lower-extremity amputation rates of minorities 50 years old or more with diabetes. J Nat Med Assoc 2005;97(3):334–8.
[7] Smith DG. Amputation. Preoperative assessment and lower extremity surgical techniques. Foot Ankle Clin 2001;6(2):271–96.

[8] Smith DG. Principles of partial foot amputations in the diabetic. AAOS Instructional Course Lectures 1999;48:321–9.
[9] Pinzur MS, Stuck RM, Sage R, et al. Syme ankle disarticulation in patients with diabetes. J Bone Joint Surg 2003;85-A(9):1667–72.
[10] Ohsawa S, Inamori Y, Fukuda K, et al. Lower limb amputation for diabetic foot. Arch Orthop Trauma Surg 2001;121:186–90.
[11] Reiber GE, Boyko EJ, Smith DG. Lower extremity foot ulcers and amputations in diabetes-National Diabetes Data Group, editors. Diabetes in America, second edition. Bethesda (MD): National Institues of Health, 1995.
[12] Weinfeld SB, Schon LC. Amputations of the perimeters of the foot. Foot Ankle Clin North Am 1999;4:17–37.
[13] Quill G, Myerson M. Clinical, radiographic, and pedobarographic analysis of the foot after hallux amputation. Presented at the American Association of Orthopedic Surgeons 58th Annual Meeting, Anaheim, CA, 1991.
[14] Lavery LA, Lavery DC, Quebedeax-Farnham TL. Increased foot pressures after greater toe amputation in diabetes. Diabetes Care 1995;18:1460–2.
[15] Graves SC, Brodie JT. Amputations below the knee. In: Mizel MS, Miller RA, Scioli MW, editors. Orthopaedic knowledge update foot and ankle 2. Rosemont (IL): American Academy of Orthopaedic Surgeons; 1998. p. 283–91.
[16] Nehler MR, Whitehill TA, Bowers SP, et al. Intermediate-term outcome of primary digit amputations in patients with diabetes mellitus who have forefoot sepsis requiring hospitalization and presumed adequate circulatory status. J Vasc Surg 1999;30(3):509–18.
[17] National Center for Health Statistics. National Hospital discharge Survey 1991. Hyattsville (MD): National Center for Health Statistics; 1993.
[18] McKittrick LS, McKittrick J, Risley TS. Transmetatarsal amputation for infection or gangrene in patients with diabetes mellitus. Ann Surg 1949;130:826–42.
[19] Sanders LJ, Dunlap G. Transmetatarsal amputation: a successful approach to limb salvage. J Am Podiatr Med Assoc 1991;82:129–35.
[20] Cohen M, Roman A, Malcolm WG. Panmetatarsal head resection and transmetatarsal amputation versus solitary partial ray resection in the neuropathic foot. J Foot Surg 1991;30:29–33.
[21] Geroulakos G, May AR. Transmetatarsal amputation in patients with peripheral vascular disease. Eur J Vasc Surg 1991;5:655–8.
[22] Thomas SRYW, Perkins JMT, Magee TR, et al. Transmetatarsal amputation: an 8-year experience. Ann R Coll Surg Engl 2001;83:164–6.
[23] Hodge MJ, Peters TG, Efird WG. Amputation of the distal portion of the foot. South Med J 1989;82:1138–42.
[24] Lynch T, Kanat IO. Transmetatarsal amputation: a literature review and case study. J Am Podiatr Med Assoc 1991;81:540–4.
[25] Miller N, Dardik H, Wolodiger F, et al. Transmetatarsal amputation: the role of adjunctive revascularization. J Vasc Surg 1991;13:705–11.
[26] Sage R, Pinzur MS, Cronin R, et al. Complications following midfoot amputation in neuropathic and dysvascular feet. J Am Podiatr Med Assoc 1989;79:277–80.
[27] Eneroth M, Apelqvist J, Larsson J, et al. Improved wound healing in transtibial amputees receiving supplementary nutrition. Int Orthop 1997;21:104–8.
[28] Lis Franc J. Nouvelle methode operatoire pour l'amputation partielle dans so articulation tarsos-metatarsienne. Paris: Sabon; 1815.
[29] Syme J. Amputation at the ankle joint. Lond Edinb Monthly J Med Sci 1843;2:93.
[30] Wagner FW Jr. Management of the diabetic-neurotrophic foot. Part II. A classification and treatment program for diabetic, neuropathic, and dysvascular foot problems. In: Cooper RR, editor. Instructional course lectures. The American Academy of Orthopaedic Surgeons. St. Louis (MO): Mosby Year Book; 1992. p. 143–65.

[31] Pinzur MS, Gottschalk F, Smith D, et al. Functional outcome of below-knee amputation in peripheral vascular insufficiency. A multicenter review. Clin Orthop 1993;286:247–9.

[32] Pinzur MS, Smith D, Osterman H. Syme ankle disarticulation in peripheral vascular disease and diabetic foot infection: the one-stage versus two-stage procedure. Foot Ankle Int 1995; 16:124–7.

[33] Bollinger M, Thordarson DB. Partial calcanectomy: an alternative to below knee amputation. Foot Ankle Int 2002;29(10):927–32.

[34] Pinzur MS. Restoration of walking ability with Syme's ankle disarticulation. Clin Orthop 1999;361:71–5.

[35] Green GV, Short K, Easley M. Transtibial amputation. Orthot Prosthet Foot Ankle 2001; 6(2):315–27.

[36] White SA, Thompson MM, Zickerman AM, et al. Lower limb amputation and grade of surgeon. Br J Surg 1997;84:509–11.

[37] Matsen SL, Malchow D, Matsen FA. Correlation with patients' perspectives of the result of lower-extremity amputation. J Bone Joint Surg 2000;82-A:1089–95.

[38] Larsson J, Agardh CD, Apelqvist J, et al. Long term prognosis after healed amputation in patients with diabetes. Clin Orthop 1998;350:149–58.

[39] Askoy DY, Gürlek A, Çetinkaya Y, et al. Change in the amputation profile in diabetic foot in a tertiary reference center: efficacy of team working. Exp Clin Endocrinol Diabetes 2004;112: 526–30.

ELSEVIER
SAUNDERS

Foot Ankle Clin N Am
11 (2006) 805–824

FOOT AND
ANKLE CLINICS

Diabetic Fracture Healing

Ankur Gandhi, PhD, Frank Liporace, MD,
Vikrant Azad, MD, James Mattie,
Sheldon S. Lin, MD*

*Department of Orthopaedics, University of Medicine & Dentistry-New Jersey Medical School,
185 South Orange Avenue, MSB G-574, Newark, NJ 07103, USA*

In the United States, more than 17 million Americans have diabetes mellitus diagnosed [1]. More than 50% of cases of diabetes are undiagnosed, and an estimated 40 million Americans will get diabetes over the next 10 years. An active lifestyle and an increase in the life expectancy of the general population also have increased the risk of fracture. The advent of improved insulin regimens or oral hyperglycemics has led to the diabetic population conforming to the general population with respect to activity and life expectancy as well as in an increase in the risk of fracture. Several clinical studies have documented the association between diabetes and impaired bone healing. Fractures in diabetic patients represent a significant challenge to the orthopedic surgeon. This review includes the few existing clinical studies documenting the effect of diabetes on bone healing (acute fractures and elective arthrodesis), preclinical studies on diabetic fracture healing, as well as specific surgical pearls and adjuncts to aid the physician in improving the clinical outcome of diabetic patients.

Clinical studies

To gain insight into the systemic effect of diabetes on bone healing, one may analyze the clinical studies regarding acute fractures and arthrodesis. A recent study of 42 ankle fracture patients evaluated complication rates among diabetic and nondiabetic patients. Those diabetic patients with other medical comorbidities have been shown to have a higher rate of complications (47%) compared with matched controls (14%). A history of Charcot

---

* Corresponding author. 90 Bergen Street, Suite 7400, DOC Building, Newark, NJ 07103.

E-mail address: linss@umdnj.edu (S.S. Lin).

1083-7515/06/$ - see front matter © 2006 Elsevier Inc. All rights reserved.
doi:10.1016/j.fcl.2006.06.009

neuroarthropathy led to the highest rates of complications in this group [2]. Cozen in 1972 suggested that diabetes mellitus affects fracture healing time [3]. In a series of 31 patients, Loder showed that time to union in diabetic patients was 163% that of nondiabetic controls. Displaced fractures in the diabetic group had the worst healing times, 187% of control [4]. A recent review of the literature and report on 80 patients with foot and ankle fractures did show that diabetics have an increased fracture healing time, 3.5 months compared with 3 months. In addition, those patients with Charcot arthropathy required at least three additional months than controls for healing [5].

Patients with sensory deficit in the foot typically have not been considered good candidates for arthrodesis due to high complication rates [6,7]. Numerous authors have reported the results of foot and ankle joints arthrodesis in patients with neuropathic arthropathy, and most have shown only limited success. Papa and colleagues [8] reported the results of open reduction and arthrodesis of various foot joints in their prospective clinical study on 29 patients with diabetic neuropathic arthropathy. The indication for the operative procedure was marked instability or a fixed deformity that could not be treated adequately with protected weight bearing. A tibiocalcaneal arthrodesis after a talectomy was attempted in 11 patients; a tibiotalar arthrodesis in eight; a triple arthrodesis in six; a tibiotalocalcaneal arthrodesis in two; and a pantalar arthrodesis in two. A pseudarthrosis developed in 10 of 29 patients (34%). However, Papa and colleagues [8] reported that in seven of those 10 cases, the pseudoarthrosis was clinically stable. There were 20 complications in 19 of the 29 patients, which included early failure of fixation in one, late fatigue failures of the screw fixation in three, superficial wound infections in three, osteomyelitis of the talus in one, wound slough in three, fractures of the distal part of the tibial diaphysis in two, malunion in two, and other soft tissue complications in five.

In a large retrospective study by Perlman and Thordarson [9] involving 88 ankle fusions, various factors that could predispose to nonunion were evaluated. Of the 67 fusions that were available for long-term follow up, 19 went on to nonunion (28%). Although a history of open injury was the only risk factor reaching statistical significance, a trend toward nonunion was seen with diabetes, smoking, illegal drug use, alcohol, and other factors. Three of the eight patients with diabetes had nonunion (38%) as compared with only 14 of 51 nondiabetic patients (27%).

Another large retrospective analysis of ankle fusion by Frey and colleagues [10] reported a high nonunion rate in patients with neurologic deficit owing to diabetes and Charcot-Marie-Tooth (CMT) disease. Clinical records and x-ray evaluation was done for a total of 78 patients with an average follow-up of 4 years. Although diabetes as a risk factor was not assessed separately, six of 12 patients with neurologic deficit had nonunion (50%).

In a retrospective evaluation of diabetic patients with peritalar neuroarthropathy undergoing triple arthrodesis, Tisdel and colleagues [11] reported the results in eight cases of arthrodesis in seven patients. Union was achieved in all eight feet demonstrable both clinically as well as radiographically. Complications included one patient with persistent wound drainage owing to *Staphylococcus aureus* infection and another with residual rocker bottom foot deformity secondary to subtalar bone resorption. All patients were reported to be satisfied with the results of surgery.

Experimental studies

Similar findings have been obtained in animal studies documenting impaired biomechanical strength of the diabetic fracture callus [12–14]. Wray and Stunkle [14] showed that the breaking strength of the healing fracture in alloxan-induced diabetic animals was significantly less than that of control animals. Herbsman and colleagues [12] found a significant reduction in the tensile strength of a fibula fracture in an alloxan-induced diabetic rat model four weeks postfracture. Macey and colleagues [13] showed that the fracture callus from the untreated animals had a 29% decrease in tensile strength and a 50% decrease in stiffness compared with nondiabetic animals 2 weeks after the production of a closed fracture.

Many inferences and an increased understanding of the fracture healing process can be obtained from data regarding the effect of diabetes on collagen synthesis and cellular proliferation. Previous studies have found decreased synthesis of collagen by articular cartilage and bone cells from diabetic rats incubated in vitro [15,16]. An additional study of collagen synthesis in cartilage cells from normal rats found that synthesis was inhibited by serum from diabetic rats [17]. Topping and colleagues [18] showed that type X collagen synthesis was decreased between 54% and 70% in the fracture callus of diabetic rats. The synthesis of type X collagen by chondrocytes undergoing hypertrophy is a critical step in the process of endochondral ossification.

Macey and colleagues [13] hypothesized that the decreased mechanical strength in the fracture callus of diabetic animals during the early stages of repair results from decreased synthesis of collagen secondary to impaired cellular proliferation or migration. Between days 4 and 11 of healing, a significant decrease (50% to 55%) in the collagen content of untreated diabetic animal fracture callus compared with controls was observed. The DNA content was decreased by 40% in the untreated diabetic group, suggesting retarded cellular proliferation. In addition, a decreased collagen to DNA ratio (representative of collagen synthesis) was documented during the 14-day healing period in diabetic animals. In comparison, the control animals showed a rapid increase in the collagen to DNA ratio as well as a rapid increase in the collagen content of the callus between days 4 and 7. The correlation of decreased mechanical strength and decreased or abnormal collagen synthesis suggests that early events play an important, persistent, and deleterious role in diabetic fracture healing.

Potential mechanisms of impaired diabetic bone healing

The mechanism through which diabetes impairs bone healing is currently unknown. The hypoinsulinemic environment associated with type I diabetes or the insulin resistance associated with type 2 diabetes both lead to a down-regulation of insulin signaling mediated through the insulin receptor. The decreased activity of the insulin signaling pathway leads to impaired glucose transport and impaired activation of critical transcription factors.

Several theories have been proposed implicating hyperglycemia and the resulting production of advanced glycation end-products as well as growth factor deficiency as major factors in diabetes-related impaired bone healing. Previous studies have shown that high glucose concentrations impair the proliferative response of osteoblastlike cells to insulinlike growth factor I (IGF-I) and delay osteoblast differentiation indicating that defective osteoblast function might contribute to impaired bone formation [19,20].

Sustained hyperglycemia increases formation of advanced glycation end products (AGEs) that can signal through a cell-surface receptor, receptor for AGE (RAGE) [21,22]. Previous studies have found that osteoblasts express RAGE and that RAGE is expressed at significantly higher levels during diabetic versus nondiabetic bone healing [21,22]. In nondiabetic animals, AGE treatment caused a dose-dependent reduction in bone healing [21,22]. These findings suggest that elevated AGE levels caused by systemic hyperglycemia contribute to diminished bone healing in diabetes, possibly mediated through RAGE.

Another possible etiology of impaired diabetic fracture healing is the role of insulin signaling on expression of specific factors critical for bone healing. In a model of intramembranous bone formation, diabetes impaired expression of Runx-2, runt domain factor-2, and Dlx5, the human homolog of the *Drosophila* distal-less gene, specific regulators of osteoblast differentiation [23]. The impaired expression of these key regulators was followed by decreased expression of osteocalcin and collagen type I corresponding to decreased bone formation measured through histomorphometric analysis. A previous fracture healing study found decreased β-fibroblastic growth factor (bFGF) expression in the early diabetic fracture callus correlated to impaired mechanical properties, which then was restored by treatment with exogenous bFGF [24]. Augmentation of bFGF stimulates fracture repair through a mitogenic effect on mesenchymal cells and through enhancement of transforming growth factor-β (TGF-β) expression, which is involved in chondrogenesis and bone formation [25–28]. Tyndall and colleagues [29] theorized that reduced platelet-derived growth factor (PDGF) expression in the early diabetic callus led to decreased cellular proliferation, which in turn resulted in impairment of the mechanical properties of the diabetic fracture callus [13].

Potential role of insulin

In 1921, Banting and Best [30] isolated insulin from the pancreas. Insulin was shown to be the major hormonal regulator of glucose metabolism and was used to treat patients who had diabetes [31]. Although the biochemistry and synthesis of insulin was not understood fully, the effects of insulin when given to diabetic patients were profound. Today, data have become available concerning insulin structure, chemistry, and its mode of action.

The primary role of insulin is to store and use glucose and other nutrients in the body, as well as inhibit glucose production [32]. Insulin activates the transporters and enzymes that are involved in the intracellular use and storage of glucose, amino acids, and fatty acids while inhibiting gluconeogenesis. Like other peptide hormones, insulin exerts its effects on cells through activation of a membrane receptor. The insulin receptor is a large transmembrane glycoprotein made up of two α and two β subunits linked by disulfide bonds. The α subunits reside outside of the cell and are responsible for insulin binding, whereas the β subunits reside intracellularly and contain the tyrosine kinase activity. Tyrosine kinase activity of the insulin receptor is initiated by insulin binding and greatly enhanced by autophosphorylation.

Although many of the details of the insulin receptor are understood, the mechanism used for downstream signaling within the cell is not known. Several possibilities exist for the intracellular pathway leading to the stimulation of glycogen synthesis and the inhibition of glyconeogenesis [32]. In addition, it is unclear how the activation of the insulin receptors leads to the translocation of a glucose transporter to allow glucose to enter the cell.

Despite the fact that the mechanism of insulin action is poorly understood, researchers are well aware of the importance of insulin in physiologic metabolic control. Type I diabetes mellitus is characterized by a complete absence of insulin secretion and an increase in circulating glucose. With the discovery of exogenous insulin treatment and tight physiologic blood glucose control, several of the long-term detrimental effects of the disease can be at least partially alleviated with insulin treatment.

In addition, insulin has been well known to have both direct and indirect action on bone. Insulin receptors have been located on rat osteoblastic cells, and insulin has been shown to stimulate proliferation in osteoblastic cells in vitro [33,34]. Insulin directly increases collagen production by osteoblasts in vitro [35]. Insulin also promotes the release of IGF-1, which stimulates both collagen synthesis and cell proliferation in osteoblasts [36,37].

Physiologic glucose control

Insulin and its association with impaired diabetic bone and mineral metabolism have been established through previous studies. Hough and colleagues [38] examined histologic parameters in intact tibiae and vertebrae of control animals as well as untreated and short- and long-term insulin-treated diabetic animals. The quantity of osteoid, epiphyseal growth plate width, and number of osteoclasts were lower in untreated diabetic animals. Insulin therapy, short- and long-term, resulted in the normalization of these histologic parameters. Diabetic animals with long-term insulin treatment had sites of bone formation and osteoclast activity that actually exceeded that of control. Verhaeghe and colleagues [39] suggested a specific role for insulin on growth plate chondrocytes and on the replication of osteoprogenitor cells. Daily infusion of insulin to diabetic rats increased the epiphyseal width of the tibiae to 30% greater than controls. Insulin treatment also increased relative surface percentages of osteoblasts, osteoclasts, osteoid tissue, and mineral apposition rate.

The timing of insulin therapy also appears to be critical. Weiss and Reddi [40] performed an analysis of ectopic bone formed with demineralized bone matrix and subsequent endochondral ossification in diabetic rats. Histologically, they noticed a delay in chondrogenesis as well as a marked reduction in vascular invasion in the diabetic plaques. The control plaques exhibited osteogenesis by day 11 and remodeling by day 14, whereas very few osteoblasts were present at day 14 in the diabetic plaques. Diabetic cell proliferation, measured by [^{3}H] thymidine uptake, reached 35% of controls at day 3 and leveled off. Injection of insulin on days 0, 1, 2, and 3, adequate to obtain physiologic blood glucose levels, increased the cell proliferation to 81% of the controls. Along with histologic features and cell proliferation, chondrogenesis was also measured by the incorporation of radioactive sulphate (^{35}S) into plaque proteoglycan on day 7. Only diabetic rats that were treated with insulin on days 0 through 7 and 0 through 4 had ^{35}SO$_4$ levels comparable with those of control animals. Animals without insulin treatment or those treated with insulin on days 3 through 7 had decreased levels of ^{35}SO$_4$ incorporation. These data suggest that the reduction of chondrogenesis may be caused by the absence of insulin during the proliferative phase of healing (days 0 through 4) leading to the decrease in cell proliferation. Mineralization, measured by incorporation of radioactive calcium-45 isotope (^{45}Ca) into the plaques, revealed less ^{45}Ca in diabetic plaques when compared with controls. When insulin was administered during the period of proliferation and chondrocyte differentiation (days 0 through 7), ^{45}Ca incorporation still was diminished. However, when insulin was administered on days 4 through 11 (representative of the osteogenesis/mineralization phase), ^{45}Ca incorporation was brought to levels not statistically different from controls. These data suggest that insulin is necessary for osteogenesis and mineralization.

The role of insulin for improving diabetic fracture healing has been analyzed in chemically induced and spontaneous diabetic rat femur fracture models [12,13,41,42]. Macey and colleagues [13] evaluated the tensile strength of the femur from normal versus untreated and insulin-treated diabetic rats 2 weeks after closed fracture. After 2 weeks, the fracture callus of untreated animals had 29% decrease in tensile strength and 50% decrease in stiffness compared with controls. In contrast, treatment of diabetic animal with insulin (despite supra-physiologic blood glucose levels) restored the tensile strength and stiffness of the callus to nonsignificant values from that of controls. Herbsman and colleagues [12] noted a similar phenomenon with the untreated diabetic rat fracture callus having reduced biomechanical properties compared with controls and insulin-treated diabetic animals.

The effects of physiologic blood glucose control on fracture healing were investigated in the diabetic rat [41]. Poorly controlled diabetic rats had decreased cell proliferation at the fracture site as well as decreased mechanical stiffness and bony content. To determine the effect of blood glucose control, diabetic rats were treated with insulin sufficient to maintain physiologic blood glucose levels throughout the course of the study. Cellular proliferation, biomechanical properties, and callus bone content in tightly controlled diabetic animals were not significantly different from nondiabetic animals. This study found that insulin treatment, resulting in improved blood glucose control, ameliorated the impaired early and late parameters of diabetic fracture healing.

To investigate the mechanisms by which insulin affects diabetes-related impaired bone formation, experiments were performed in a marrow ablation model that mimics intramembranous bone formation [23]. Insulin treatment substantially reversed the effect of diabetes on the expression of bone matrix osteocalcin and collagen type I and osteoblast transcription factors Runx2 and Dlx5. These results indicate that diabetic animals produce sufficient amounts of immature mesenchymal tissue but fail to adequately express genes that regulate osteoblast differentiation leading to decreased bone formation.

Local delivery of factors

Few studies have explored the effect of locally applied growth factor on normal osseous and diabetic fracture healing. Kirkeby and Ekeland [43] delivered IGF-1 locally by an osmotic pump (100 μg per 100 g body weight daily) into the rat femoral osteotomy model as described previously. No significant difference was noted compared with control (saline vehicle only) with regard to torsional strength, deformation, stiffness, radiographic healing, callus weight, or callus mineralization . In contrast, other in vivo studies have shown that local application of IGF-1 using pumps and catheters have a positive effect on fracture healing [44,45].

Schmidmaier and colleagues [46,47] evaluated the synergistic effect of locally delivered growth factors (IGF-I and TGF-β1) using a biodegradable poly(D,L-lactide)-coated osteosynthesis implant in Sprague Dawley rat tibial fracture model. Comparison of callus morphology and proliferation rate showed differences during fracture healing owing to the local application of IGF-I and TGF-β1 from coated implants [48]. Biomechanical testing found a significant higher maximum load and torsional stiffness; histologic/

histomorphometric analysis showed progressive remodeling after 28 and 42 days in the group treated with growth factors compared with controls. These findings suggest that the local application of growth factors from local intramedullary systems accelerates fracture healing [46,47]. Raschke and colleagues [49] reported similar findings, using a similar IGF-1– and TGF-β1–coated implant in an osteotomy model of minipigs. Currently, it remains unclear what stages of the repair process are influenced by the locally administered IGF-I.

Diabetic fracture healing adjuncts

Few studies exist regarding the effect of local fracture healing adjuncts in a diabetic animal model (Table 1). These studies include the use of low-intensity pulsed ultrasound (US), biodegradable microcapsules containing bone formation stimulant (TAK-778), recombinant human bFGF, local delivery of insulin, and the percutaneous injection of platelet-rich plasma (PRP) [24,50–53]. US normalized the diabetes-related impairment in fracture callus strength [52]; however, US did not affect cellular proliferation in the early diabetic fracture callus. The effect of US in a diabetic fracture healing model does not appear to be mediated through the normalization of cell number but possibly through increased matrix production. Hoshino and colleagues [53] reported locally delivered microcapsules of TAK-778–enhanced fracture repair in streptozotocin-induced diabetic rats. TAK-778 increased the bending strength of diabetic bone at 4 weeks and 8 weeks. The fracture callus was remodeled, and cortical bony union was demonstrated in the TAK-778–treated diabetic group compared with the fibrous nonunion in diabetic-only group. Kawaguchi and colleagues [24] found decreased levels of bFGF in the diabetic rat fibula fracture callus, which was restored to normal values under physiologic insulin treatment. The exogenous application of rhFGF increased levels of TGF-β at the fracture site in diabetic rats as well as restored the volume and mineral content of diabetic callus.

Gandhi and colleagues [50,51] showed in a diabetic femur fracture model that diabetes impairs the fracture healing process beginning with a reduction in early cellular proliferation, continuing with a delay in endochondral ossification and ending with a decrease in the biomechanical properties of the fracture callus. These impairments seem to occur secondary to reductions in insulin and certain mitogenic and osteogenic growth factors. A novel intramedullary insulin delivery system was used to investigate the potential direct effects of insulin on bone healing [50]. Insulin delivery at the fracture site normalized the early and late parameters of diabetic fracture healing without affecting the systemic parameters of blood glucose. These results suggest a critical role for insulin in directly mediating fracture healing and that decreased systemic insulin levels in the diabetic state lead to reduced

Table 1
Diabetic fracture healing adjuncts

Study	Year	Treatment	Model	Results
Kawaguchi et al [40]	1994	Recombinant human basic fibroblast growth factor (rhbFGF)	Rat fibula fracture	Local application of rhbFGF increases the volume and mineral content in a dose-dependent manner and normalizes diabetic callus formation.
Hoshino et al [33]	2000	TAK-778	Rat fibula fracture	TAK-778 normalizes diabetic callus formation and significantly improves the biomechanical strength of the diabetic fracture callus.
Beam et al [4]	2002	Systemic insulin	Rat femur fracture	'Physiologic blood glucose control' normalizes the early and late parameters of diabetic fracture healing.
Gebauer et al [28]	2002	US	Rat femur fracture	US significantly improved biomechanical properties of the diabetic fracture callus without affecting early cell proliferation.
Follak et al [20]	2005	Systemic insulin	Rat femur fracture	"Physiologic blood glucose control" normalizes the histomorphometric and biomechanical parameters of diabetic fracture healing.
Gandhi et al [23]	2005	Local insulin	Rat femur fracture	Local insulin delivery normalizes the early and late parameters of diabetic fracture healing without affecting systemic blood glucose levels.
Gandhi et al [24]	2005	PRP	Rat femur fracture	PRP normalizes the early parameters of diabetic fracture healing and significantly improves the biomechanical strength of the diabetic fracture callus.

localized insulin levels at the fracture site with concomitant increases in diabetic fracture healing time. Treatment with PRP, however, does not lead to a normalization of the diabetic fracture healing environment but does correct for the growth factor–deficient environment present at the site of injury in the early diabetic callus [51]. Ameliorating impaired growth factor expression within the diabetic fracture site normalizes the early cell proliferation and cartilage formation but only partially restores the biomechanical strength of the healing fracture. These results suggest a role for PRP in mediating diabetic fracture healing and potentially other high-risk fractures.

Treatment of ankle fractures in diabetics

General overview

Patients with diabetes and ankle fractures represent a subset of the population that historically has been viewed as difficult to treat with increased complication rates. As with all fractures, non-operative and operative indications exist. All diabetic ankle fracture patients need to be informed of potential increased complications (wound healing problems, deep infection delayed/nonunion) [2,5,54–59]. Tight blood glucose control remains important in avoiding complications and improving outcomes [54].

A recent review of 160,598 patients, from the Nationwide Inpatient Sample database of patients treated for ankle fractures from 1988 through 2000, showed that 9714 (5.71%) patients treated had diabetes mellitus. Those patients with diabetes had a significantly greater in-hospital mortality, rate of in-hospital postoperative complications, length of hospital stay, total charges, and rate of nonroutine discharge. This held true for all levels of fracture severity (closed, unimalleolar, closed bimalleolar or trimalleolar, and dislocated or open fractures) [60].

Nonoperative treatment

Nonoperative treatment involves casting with weight-bearing restrictions. Typically, immobilization and non–weight bearing are done for durations of two to three times that of nondiabetic patients in an effort to avoid malunion and Charcot arthropathy [2,54]. Although less common in the ankle, Charcot arthropathy can develop as a posttraumatic event [54,56,61]. Therefore, one paramount test is to evaluate diabetic patients for sensory deficits, with a 5.07 SW monofilament. Patients with pre-existing neuropathy are at an increased risk of unrecognized microtrauma that can result in such complications [54,56,61].

Closed treatment does not bar a patient from the risk of infection. In a recent series of 98 closed ankle fractures, the overall infection rate was 32% in the diabetic population compared with 8% in the nondiabetic population [54]. Infection in the surgically treated group of diabetics was more than double that in the surgically treated nondiabetics. Also, infection developed in four of six diabetic patients treated in a closed manner compared with no infection seen in the five nondiabetics treated by closed means. In those diabetics treated surgically, the infection rate was only four of 19 patients. Noncompliance with diabetes treatment, peripheral vascular disease, peripheral neuropathy, swelling, and ecchymosis increased the risk for infection in the diabetic population [57].

Connolly and Csencsitz [56] reported on six diabetic patients with low-energy ankle twisting injuries. Of the five patients treated nonoperatively, all had complications including infection, nonunion, malunion, and posttraumatic arthrosis. One case resulted in amputation. Sensory neuropathies increased the risk of ulcerations, infections, and posttraumatic deformities from unprotected weight bearing on the insensate foot.

Operative fixation

Operative treatment of ankle fractures in diabetics also holds a concerning rate of complications. In a review of 67 patients with ankle fractures (21 with diabetes), the complication rate among the diabetics was 43% compared with 15.5% in the nondiabetic group. Complications in the diabetics included five deep infections, three losses of fixation, and two below-knee amputations [55]. Another recent review of 26 diabetic and 26 nondiabetic patients with ankle fractures had 42.3% versus 0% complication rates, respectively. Among the diabetic patients treated operatively, six (31.6%) had postoperative complications. There was one malunion, one wound edge necrosis requiring a flap, two cases of deep sepsis, and two below-knee amputations eventually resulting in death [58]. Low and Tan [62] reviewed 93 patients, 10 with diabetes, treated operatively for ankle fractures. Of the five patients in the series with wound infections, all five (100%) had diabetes mellitus. Two of these patients eventually required a below-knee amputation.

One recent series looked specifically at open ankle fractures in patients with diabetes [59]. Fourteen open ankle fractures were identified in 13 patients with a mean follow-up of 19 months. The need for additional surgical procedures and number of complications were high. The average number of surgical procedures per patient was five. Nine extremities had wound healing complications. Five cases ultimately resulted in below-knee amputations. Only three patients (21%) had uneventful healing without complications [59].

Although multiple options for internal fixation exist, before performing open surgery, soft-tissue stabilization is paramount. Bibbo and colleagues [54] has stressed the importance of a treatment protocol that involves prompt reduction and splinting to reduce soft tissue trauma, delayed surgery for resolution of edema, and medical optimization before formal open reduction and internal fixation. To maintain reduction while pending soft tissue stabilization, external fixation may be necessary and can be combined with internal fixation based on the ultimate condition of the soft tissue envelope [63].

Surgical technique: pearls

Operatively indicated fractures in diabetic patients require very rigid fixation to avoid complications. External fixation may need to be used acutely for a staged plating or as definitive treatment if severe concomitant soft tissue injury is present. Osteoporosis also is a frequent concern when dealing with these patients; therefore, supplementation to standard ankle fixation commonly is required. To increase rigidity of fixation, longer plates, supplementary k-wires in plated fibulas, multiple fibula-tibia syndesmotic fixation, and transcalcaneal-tibial Steinmann pin fixation all have been suggested as adjuncts to standard surgical options [64–68]. The use of locked plating may provide the added stability, in cases of severe bone loss and comminution commonly seen with these patients. Also, percutaneous fibula fixation may be considered to avoid wound complications [69].

Sanders and colleagues [68] have hypothesized that longer plates with minimum numbers of screws provide equivalent or superior strength of fixation to standard compression plating using the maximum number of screws. The investigators used a cadaveric model comparing fixation with six, eight, or 10-hole plates with two screws at the outermost holes and two screws at the innermost holes to fracture fixation with a six-hole plate with all screw-holes filled. The eight-hole plate with only four screws was as rigid as the six-hole plate with six screws. Additionally, the rigidity of the construct was increased based on the length of the plate. Therefore, the number of screws is less important than the length of the plate in providing bending strength to a construct.

Koval and colleagues [66] has suggested a method for increasing purchase of screws during fibula plate fixation in osteoporotic bone. First retrograde 1.6-mm k-wires are placed across a reduced distal fibula fracture and penetrate the fibula's medial cortex in the proximal fragment. Then a precontoured one-third tubular plate is applied to the lateral aspect of the fibula with its screws interdigitating with the intramedullary retrograde k-wires (Fig. 1). In 19 patients with an average 15.4-month follow-up, 89% had either no pain, slight, or mild pain. When biomechanically comparing this mode of fixation to standard fibula plating, the specimens augmented with k-wires had 81% greater resistance to bending and twice the resistance to motion during torsional testing.

In an effort to further improve fixation stiffness on the augmented k-wire model, Dunn and colleagues [64] and Schon and Marks [63] used multiple tetra-cortical fibula-to-tibia screw fixation through the one-third tubular plate in the proximal fibula fragment, in addition to intramedullary k-wire fixation (Fig. 2). Biomechanically, when comparing the intramedullary k-wire supplemented fixation to a similar construct with the addition of three tetra-cortical syndesmotic screws, the later construct was significantly stiffer in resisting axial and external rotation loads [64]. A recent series of six patients, with failed neuropathic ankle fractures, used a similar technique with the addition of a 4.5-mm dynamic compression plate (DCP) plate and multiple 4.5-mm tetra-cortical syndesmotic screws [67].

The use of fibula-to-tibia tetra-cortical screws has been suggested to alter the biomechanics of the ankle by changing the stiffness of the syndesmosis, specifically decreasing in tibiotalar external rotation and anterior-posterior draw in plantar flexion. One major concern of this technique is the potential for screw breakage [70]. Clinically, this concern has been shown to not be significant because ambulation progressively restores motion between the tibia and fibula in spite of fixation as evidenced by lysis around syndesmotic screws [71].

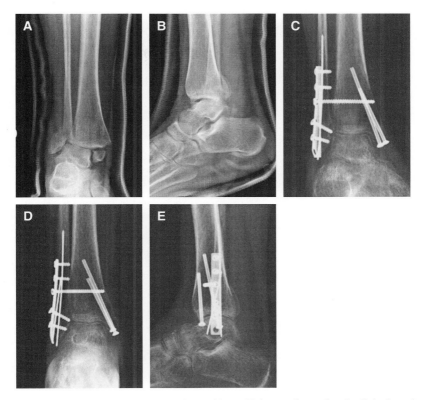

Fig. 1. (*A, B*) Preoperative antero-posterior and lateral injury radiographs of a diabetic patient with a trimalleolar ankle fracture/subluxation. (*C, D, E*) Postoperative anterior-posterior, mortise, and lateral radiographs of the same patient after using supplementary intramedullary fibula kirschner wires combined with a standard lateral plating of the fibula and medial malleolar screw fixation.

The introduction of locked plating may help with attaining stable fixation. Fixed angle screws do not rely on friction between the plate and bone; therefore, failure requires "cutting-out" of all the points of fixation on one side of the fracture as opposed to loosening of individual screws resulting in localized failure of the construct as is seen with traditional plating. Recent biomechanical studies have found that locked fixation is better at retaining its original stiffness compared with traditional plating when subjected to cyclical loading [72,73]. To date, no long-term studies of ankle fracture fixation have been evaluated with locked plating.

In patients with unstable ankle fractures and loss of protective sensibility confirmed via testing with a 5.07 Semmes-Weinstein monofilament, transarticular fixation and prolonged, protected weight bearing has been suggested as a viable treatment option [65]. To improve construct rigidity in 15 diabetics with 16 ankle fractures and deficient protective sensation, retrograde

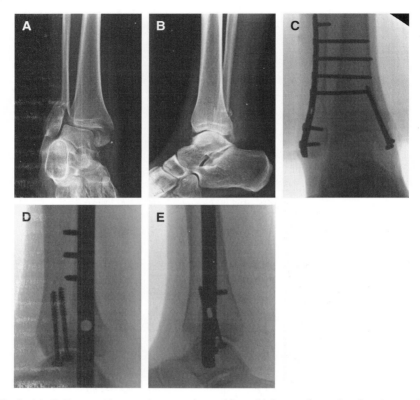

Fig. 2. (*A, B*) Preoperative anterior-posterior and lateral injury radiographs of a 19-year-old man with a 12-year history of insulin dependent diabetes mellitus (IDDM) who sustained a bimalleolar ankle fracture/subluxation. (*C, D, E*) Postoperative anterior-posterior, and lateral radiographs (ankle joint lateral and lateral in the plane of the three superior syndesmotic screws) of the same patient after using tetracortical syndesmotic screw supplementary fixation with a fibula plating and medial malleolar screw fixation. Distally, in this severely osteoporotic patient, locked screws were used in the one-third tubular locking plate because the patient's fibula intramedullary diameter and geometry were not optimal for supplementary intramedullary k-wire fixation.

transcalcaneal-talar-tibial fixation using large Steinmann pins or screws in conjunction with standard techniques of open reduction and internal fixation were used. Postoperatively, patients were placed in a short leg, total contact cast and made non–weight bearing for 12 weeks. Removal of the intramedullary implants took place at 12 to 16 weeks. Then patients were placed in a walking boot or cast with partial weigh bearing for an additional 12 weeks. Finally, patients were transitioned to a custom-molded, ankle-foot orthosis or custom total-contact inserts. Major complication rate for all fractures was 25%. Of the closed fractures, one of 13 went on to amputation. There were no deaths or Charcot malunions in the series [65].

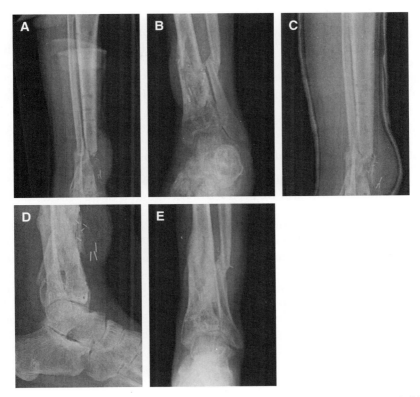

Fig. 3. (*A, B*) Preoperative antero-posterior and lateral view of the left ankle shows distal tibial nonunion. (*C*) Fourteen-day postoperative bone grafting with Symphony Platelet Concentration Systems (PCS) shows early callus formation. (*D*) Twenty-eight–day postoperative bone grafting with Symphony PCS shows more callus formation. (*E, F*) Two-year follow-up antero-posterior, mortise, and lateral view of the left ankle shows healed nonunion.

To avoid large incisions and to decrease wound healing complications, percutaneous fibula fixation may be attempted in closed, low-energy, non-comminuted, length-stable fibula fractures. This may be done with either a plate or intramedullary screw. Through a limited incision distally, a pre-contoured small fragment plate can be advanced retrograde along the lateral aspect of the fibula to the appropriate level with the aid of orthogonal fluoroscopy. Percutaneous, provisional proximal and distal fixation of the plate can be accomplished with k-wires through the most proximal and distal plate holes. Next, through small incisions, screw fixation can be applied through the plate to the proximal and distal fragments. This technique does not preclude tetracortical syndesmotic fixation, which may be necessary to improve the biomechanical characteristics of the construct.

In a truly transverse fracture, percutaneous intramedullary fixation of the lateral malleolus with a retrograde screw can be done [69]. Once closed fracture reduction is confirmed with fluoroscopy, a guidewire for a fully threaded self-tapping screw can be inserted through a small incision just distal to the lateral malleolus. A cannulated drill can be inserted over the guidewire and exchanged for a self-tapping screw after drilling is complete. Screw diameter is based on the patient's anatomy. If the fracture is not rotationally stable, the screw can be placed bicortically through the medial fibular cortex in the proximal fragment.

Potential for patient with diabetes to develop a fracture

Progressive microvascular disease in diabetes can lead to decreased blood flow peripherally. Progressive decrease in perfusion to the lower extremities of patients has been shown to negatively affect bone mineral density. Those with marked decrease in annual blood flow have a larger annual rate of bone loss than those with relatively stable blood flow [74]. Bone mineral density can affect the type of injury experienced by a diabetic patient with neuropathic arthropathy. A review of 55 diabetic patients with foot and ankle trauma showed that if osteopenia was present, the odds ratio of development of fracture as opposed to a dislocation was 9.5 [75]. Patients with diabetes have been shown to have an increased rate of sustaining more severe ankle fractures than patients without diabetes (Fig. 3.) [60].

Summary

Patients with diabetic ankle fractures consistently are at greater risk of sustaining a complication during treatment than nondiabetics. Other medical comorbidities, especially Charcot neuroarthropathy and peripheral vascular disease, play distinct roles in increasing these complication rates. Many options for nonoperative and operative treatment exist, but respect for soft tissue management and attention to stable, rigid fixation with prolonged immobilization and prolonged restricted weight bearing are paramount in trying to minimize problems and yield functional results.

Further readings

Bibbo C. Autologous platelet concentrate in high-risk foot & ankle surgery. Presented at the AOFAS 20th Annual Summer Meeting. Seattle, July 14, 2004.

Bibbo C, Bono CM, Lin SS. Union rates using autologous platelet concentrate alone and with bone graft in high-risk foot and ankle surgery patients. J Surg Orthop Adv 2005;14:17–22.

Cmolik BL, Spero JA, Magovern GJ, et al. Redo cardiac surgery: late bleeding complications from topical thrombin-induced factor V deficiency. J Thorac Cardiovasc Surg 1993;105: 222–7 [discussion: 227–8].

Coetzee J, Bono CM, Lin SS. The use of autologous concentrated growth factors to promote syndesmosis fusion in the agility total ankle replacement: a preliminary study. Foot Ankle Int 2005;26(10):840–6.

Coetzee J, Pometroy G, Watts D, et al. The use of autologous concentrated growth factors in fusion rates in the agility total ankle replacement: a preliminary study. Presented at the AOFAS 20th Annual Summer Meeting. Seattle, July 14, 2004.

Efeoglu C, Akcay YD, Erturk S. A modified method for preparing platelet-rich plasma: an experimental study. J Oral Maxillofac Surg 2004;62:1403–7.

Gandhi A, Van Gelderen J, Berberian WS, et al. Platelet releasate enhances healing in patients with a non-union. Presented at the Orthopaedic Research Society 49th Annual Meeting. New Orleans, Louisiana, February 20, 2003.

Landesberg R, Moses M, Karpatkin M. Risks of using platelet rich plasma gel. J Oral Maxillofac Surg 1998;56:1116–7.

Landesberg R, Roy M, Glickman RS. Quantification of growth factor levels using a simplified method of platelet-rich plasma gel preparation. J Oral Maxillofac Surg 2000;58:297–300 [discussion: 300–1].

References

[1] Lee TH. Diabetic foot. In: M. Mizel, editor. OKU foot & ankle 1. Rosemont (IL): American Academy of Orthopaedic Surgeons; 1996.

[2] Jones KB, Maiers-Yelden KA, Marsh JL, et al. Ankle fractures in patients with diabetes mellitus. J Bone Joint Surg Br 2005;87:489–95.

[3] Cozen L. Does diabetes delay fracture healing? Clin Orthop 1972;82:134–40.

[4] Loder RT. The influence of diabetes mellitus on the healing of closed fractures. Clin Orthop 1988;232:210–6.

[5] Boddenberg U. Healing time of foot and ankle fractures in patients with diabetes mellitus: literature review and report on own cases. Zentralbl Chir 2004;129:453–9 [in German].

[6] Johnson EW Jr. The surgical management of diabetic complications. W V Med J 1958;54: 157–61.

[7] Ouzounian TJ, Kleiger B. Arthrodesis in foot and ankle. In: Jahss ML, editor. Disorders of the foot. Philadelphia: W.B. Saunders; 1988.

[8] Papa J, Myerson M, Girard P. Salvage, with arthrodesis, in intractable diabetic neuropathic arthropathy of the foot and ankle. J Bone Joint Surg Am 1993;75:1056–66.

[9] Perlman MH, Thordarson DB. Ankle fusion in a high risk population: an assessment of nonunion risk factors. Foot Ankle Int 1999;20:491–6.

[10] Frey C, Halikus NM, Vu-Rose T, et al. A review of ankle arthrodesis: predisposing factors to nonunion. Foot Ankle Int 1994;15:581–4.

[11] Tisdel CL, Marcus RE, Heiple KG. Triple arthrodesis for diabetic peritalar neuroarthropathy. Foot Ankle Int 1995;16:332–8.

[12] Herbsman H, Powers JC, Hirschman A, et al. Retardation of fracture healing in experimental diabetes. J Surg Res 1968;8:424–31.

[13] Macey LR, Kana SM, Jingushi S, et al. Defects of early fracture-healing in experimental diabetes. J Bone Joint Surg Am 1989;71:722–33.

[14] Wray JB, Stunkle E. The effect of experimental diabetes upon the breaking strength of the healing fracture in the rat. J Surg Res 1965;5:479–81.

[15] Spanheimer RG. Direct inhibition of collagen production in vitro by diabetic rat serum. Metabolism 1988;37:479–85.

[16] Spanheimer RG, Umpierrez GE, Stumpf V. Decreased collagen production in diabetic rats. Diabetes 1988;37:371–6.

[17] Spanheimer RG. Correlation between decreased collagen production in diabetic animals and in cells exposed to diabetic serum: response to insulin. Matrix 1992;12:101–7.

[18] Topping RE, Bolander ME, Balian G. Type X collagen in fracture callus and the effects of experimental diabetes. Clin Orthop 1994;308:220–8.

[19] Balint E, Szabo P, Marshall CF, et al. Glucose-induced inhibition of in vitro bone mineralization. Bone 2001;28:21–8.

[20] Terada M, Inaba M, Yano Y, et al. Growth-inhibitory effect of a high glucose concentration on osteoblast-like cells. Bone 1998;22:17–23.

[21] Cortizo AM, Lettieri MG, Barrio DA, et al. Advanced glycation end-products (AGEs) induce concerted changes in the osteoblastic expression of their receptor RAGE and in the activation of extracellular signal-regulated kinases (ERK). Mol Cell Biochem 2003; 250:1–10.

[22] Santana RB, Xu L, Chase HB, et al. A role for advanced glycation end products in diminished bone healing in type 1 diabetes. Diabetes 2003;52:1502–10.

[23] Lu H, Kraut D, Gerstenfeld LC, et al. Diabetes interferes with the bone formation by affecting the expression of transcription factors that regulate osteoblast differentiation. Endocrinology 2003;144:346–52.

[24] Kawaguchi H, Kurokawa T, Hanada K, et al. Stimulation of fracture repair by recombinant human basic fibroblast growth factor in normal and streptozotocin-diabetic rats. Endocrinology 1994;135:774–81.

[25] Joyce ME, Jingushi S, Bolander ME. Transforming growth factor-beta in the regulation of fracture repair. Orthop Clin North Am 1990;21:199–209.

[26] McCarthy TL, Centrella M, Canalis E. Effects of fibroblast growth factors on deoxyribonucleic acid and collagen synthesis in rat parietal bone cells. Endocrinology 1989;125: 2118–26.

[27] Noda M, Camilliere JJ. In vivo stimulation of bone formation by transforming growth factor-beta. Endocrinology 1989;124:2991–4.

[28] Noda M, Vogel R. Fibroblast growth factor enhances type beta 1 transforming growth factor gene expression in osteoblast-like cells. J Cell Biol 1989;109:2529–35.

[29] Tyndall WA, Beam HA, Zarro C, et al. Decreased platelet derived growth factor expression during fracture healing in diabetic animals. Clin Orthop 2003;403:319–30.

[30] Banting FG, Best CH. The internal secretion of the pancreas. J Lab Clin Med 1922;7:251–66.

[31] Banting FG, Best CH, Collip JB, et al. Pancreatic extracts in the treatment of diabetes mellitus: preliminary report. 1922. CMAJ 1991;145:1281–6.

[32] White MF, Kahn CR. Molecular aspects of insulin action. In: Kahn CR, Weir GC, editors. Joslin's diabetes mellitus. 13th edition. Philadelphia: Lea and Febiger; 1994. p. 139–62.

[33] Hickman J, McElduff A. Insulin promotes growth of the cultured rat osteosarcoma cell line UMR-106–01: an osteoblast-like cell. Endocrinology 1989;124:701–6.

[34] Levy JR, Murray E, Manolagas S, et al. Demonstration of insulin receptors and modulation of alkaline phosphatase activity by insulin in rat osteoblastic cells. Endocrinology 1986;119: 1786–92.

[35] Gabbitas B, Pash J, Canalis E. Regulation of insulin-like growth factor-II synthesis in bone cell cultures by skeletal growth factors. Endocrinology 1994;135:284–9.

[36] Einhorn TA, Boskey AL, Gundberg CM, et al. The mineral and mechanical properties of bone in chronic experimental diabetes. J Orthop Res 1988;6:317–23.

[37] Machwate M, Zerath E, Holy X, et al. Insulin-like growth factor-I increases trabecular bone formation and osteoblastic cell proliferation in unloaded rats. Endocrinology 1994;134:1031–8.

[38] Hough S, Avioli LV, Bergfeld MA, et al. Correction of abnormal bone and mineral metabolism in chronic streptozotocin-induced diabetes mellitus in the rat by insulin therapy. Endocrinology 1981;108:2228–34.

[39] Verhaeghe J, Suiker AM, Visser WJ, et al. The effects of systemic insulin, insulin-like growth factor-I and growth hormone on bone growth and turnover in spontaneously diabetic BB rats. J Endocrinol 1992;134:485–92.

[40] Weiss RE, Reddi AH. Influence of experimental diabetes and insulin on matrix-induced cartilage and bone differentiation. Am J Physiol 1980;238:E200–7.

[41] Beam HA, Parsons JR, Lin SS. The effects of blood glucose control upon fracture healing in the BB Wistar rat with diabetes mellitus. J Orthop Res 2002;20:1210–6.

[42] Follak N, Kloting I, Merk H. Influence of diabetic metabolic state on fracture healing in spontaneously diabetic rats. Diabetes Metab Res Rev 2005;21:288–96.

[43] Kirkeby OJ, Ekeland A. No effects of local somatomedin C on bone repair. Continuous infusion in rats. Acta Orthop Scand 1992;63:447–50.

[44] Isgaard J, Nilsson A, Lindahl A, et al. Effects of local administration of GH and IGF-1 on longitudinal bone growth in rats. Am J Physiol 1986;250:E367–72.

[45] Nielsen HM, Andreassen TT, Ledet T, et al. Local injection of TGF-beta increases the strength of tibial fractures in the rat. Acta Orthop Scand 1994;65:37–41.

[46] Schmidmaier G, Wildemann B, Bail H, et al. Local application of growth factors (insulin-like growth factor-1 and transforming growth factor-beta1) from a biodegradable poly(D,L-lactide) coating of osteosynthetic implants accelerates fracture healing in rats. Bone 2001;28:341–50.

[47] Schmidmaier G, Wildemann B, Gabelein T, et al. Synergistic effect of IGF-I and TGF-beta1 on fracture healing in rats: single versus combined application of IGF-I and TGF-beta1. Acta Orthop Scand 2003;74:604–10.

[48] Wildemann B, Schmidmaier G, Ordel S, et al. Cell proliferation and differentiation during fracture healing are influenced by locally applied IGF-I and TGF-beta1: comparison of two proliferation markers, PCNA and BrdU. J Biomed Mater Res 2003;65B:150–6.

[49] Raschke M, Wildemann B, Inden P, et al. Insulin-like growth factor-1 and transforming growth factor-beta1 accelerates osteotomy healing using polylactide-coated implants as a delivery system: a biomechanical and histological study in minipigs. Bone 2002;30:144–51.

[50] Gandhi A, Beam HA, O'Connor JP, et al. The effects of local insulin delivery on diabetic fracture healing. Bone 2005;37:482–90.

[51] Gandhi A, Dumas C, O'Connor JP, et al. The effects of local platelet rich plasma delivery on diabetic fracture healing. Bone 2005;38(4):540–6.

[52] Gebauer GP, Lin SS, Beam HA, et al. Low-intensity pulsed ultrasound increases the fracture callus strength in diabetic BB Wistar rats but does not affect cellular proliferation. J Orthop Res 2002;20:587–92.

[53] Hoshino T, Muranishi H, Saito K, et al. Enhancement of fracture repair in rats with streptozotocin-induced diabetes by a single injection of biodegradable microcapsules containing a bone formation stimulant, TAK-778. J Biomed Mater Res 2000;51:299–306.

[54] Bibbo C, Lin SS, Beam HA, et al. Complications of ankle fractures in diabetic patients. Orthop Clin North Am 2001;32:113–33.

[55] Blotter RH, Connolly E, Wasan A, et al. Acute complications in the operative treatment of isolated ankle fractures in patients with diabetes mellitus. Foot Ankle Int 1999;20:687–94.

[56] Connolly JF, Csencsitz TA. Limb threatening neuropathic complications from ankle fractures in patients with diabetes. Clin Orthop Relat Res 1998;March(348):212–9.

[57] Flynn JM, Rodriguez-del Rio F, Piza PA. Closed ankle fractures in the diabetic patient. Foot Ankle Int 2000;21:311–9.

[58] McCormack RG, Leith JM. Ankle fractures in diabetics. Complications of surgical management. J Bone Joint Surg Br 1998;80:689–92.

[59] White CB, Turner NS, Lee GC, et al. Open ankle fractures in patients with diabetes mellitus. Clin Orthop Relat Res 2003;Sept(414):37–44.

[60] Ganesh SP, Pietrobon R, Cecilio WA, et al. The impact of diabetes on patient outcomes after ankle fracture. J Bone Joint Surg Am 2005;87:1712–8.

[61] Graves M, Tarquinio TA. Diabetic neuroarthropathy (Charcot joints): the importance of recognizing chronic sensory deficits in the treatment of acute foot and ankle fractures in diabetic patients. Orthopedics 2003;26:415–8.

[62] Low CK, Tan SK. Infection in diabetic patients with ankle fractures. Ann Acad Med Singapore 1995;24:353–5.

[63] Schon LC, Marks RM. The management of neuroarthropathic fracture-dislocations in the diabetic patient. Orthop Clin North Am 1995;26:375–92.

[64] Dunn WR, Easley ME, Parks BG, et al. An augmented fixation method for distal fibular fractures in elderly patients: a biomechanical evaluation. Foot Ankle Int 2004;25:128–31.

[65] Jani MM, Ricci WM, Borrelli J Jr, et al. A protocol for treatment of unstable ankle fractures using transarticular fixation in patients with diabetes mellitus and loss of protective sensibility. Foot Ankle Int 2003;24:838–44.

[66] Koval KJ, Petraco DM, Kummer FJ, et al. A new technique for complex fibula fracture fixation in the elderly: a clinical and biomechanical evaluation. J Orthop Trauma 1997;11:28–33.

[67] Perry MD, Taranow WS, Manoli A 2nd, et al. Salvage of failed neuropathic ankle fractures: use of large-fragment fibular plating and multiple syndesmotic screws. J Surg Orthop Adv 2005;14:85–91.

[68] Sanders R, Haidukewych GJ, Milne T, et al. Minimal versus maximal plate fixation techniques of the ulna: the biomechanical effect of number of screws and plate length. J Orthop Trauma 2002;16:166–71.

[69] Ray TD, Nimityongskul P, Anderson LD. Percutaneous intramedullary fixation of lateral malleolus fractures: technique and report of early results. J Trauma 1994;36:669–75.

[70] Needleman RL, Skrade DA, Stiehl JB. Effect of the syndesmotic screw on ankle motion. Foot Ankle 1989;10:17–24.

[71] Kaye RA. Stabilization of ankle syndesmosis injuries with a syndesmosis screw. Foot Ankle 1989;9:290–3.

[72] Gardner MJ, Brophy RH, Campbell D, et al. The mechanical behavior of locking compression plates compared with dynamic compression plates in a cadaver radius model. J Orthop Trauma 2005;19:597–603.

[73] Liporace FA, Gupta S, Jeong GK, et al. A biomechanical comparison of a dorsal 3.5-mm T-plate and a volar fixed-angle plate in a model of dorsally unstable distal radius fractures. J Orthop Trauma 2005;19:187–91.

[74] Vogt MT, Cauley JA, Kuller LH, et al. Bone mineral density and blood flow to the lower extremities: the study of osteoporotic fractures. J Bone Miner Res 1997;12:283–9.

[75] Herbst SA, Jones KB, Saltzman CL. Pattern of diabetic neuropathic arthropathy associated with the peripheral bone mineral density. J Bone Joint Surg Br 2004;86:378–83.

ELSEVIER
SAUNDERS

Foot Ankle Clin N Am
11 (2006) 825–835

FOOT AND
ANKLE CLINICS

Charcot of the Calcaneus

Lucille B. Andersen, MD[a], John DiPreta, MD[b],*

[a]Department of Orthopaedics and Rehabilitation, Penn State Milton S. Hershey Medical
Center, 500 University Drive, P.O. Box 850, H089, Hershey, PA 17033-0850, USA
[b]Division of Orthopaedic Surgery, Department of Surgery, Albany Medical Center,
Mail code 184, Albany, NY 12208, USA

Charcot arthropathy of the calcaneus presents difficulty on numerous levels for the orthopedist. The paucity of literature and research regarding treatment and outcome leaves many practitioners adrift. The basis of treatment primarily relies on information gleaned about Charcot in different joints.

Jean Martin Charcot first described neuroarthropathy in 1868 as it pertained to patients with tabes dorsalis [1]. There is a plethora of causes of Charcot joints including spina bifida, meningomyelocele, thalidomide ingestion, spinal cord trauma, polio, transverse myelitis, cystic disease of bone, congenital indifference to pain, familiar dysautonomia, progressive sensory neuropathy, spinal cord tumor, spinal dysraphism, and amyloid neuropathy [2]. The top four causes are tabes, leprosy, syringomyelia, and diabetes mellitus [2]. It was not until 1936 that Jordan reported on neuropathic arthropathy in patients with diabetes mellitus [3,4]. Bailey described the painless destruction of the tarsus in 14 patients with uncontrolled diabetes in 1942 [3]. One of the few reports to mention calcaneal Charcot exclusively was not published until 1979. Coventry and Rothacker [5] noted an incidence of bilateral atraumatic calcaneus fractures in a patient with diabetes and neuropathic changes. Where these types of injuries were once notable as case studies, now that modern insulin therapy has greatly increased the longevity of patients with diabetes, they are becoming more prevalent.

It is estimated that 25% of Medicare expenditure is directed toward management of patients with diabetes mellitus. Five percent of health care dollars is consumed in the management of the complications secondary to diabetes [6]. In 1996 it was estimated that there were 16 million patients in the United States with diabetes mellitus [7]. The incidence of Charcot

* Corresponding author.
E-mail address: jamddipreta@netscape.net (J. DiPreta).

1083-7515/06/$ - see front matter © 2006 Elsevier Inc. All rights reserved.
doi:10.1016/j.fcl.2006.06.010

foot.theclinics.com

in patients with diabetes is estimated to be anywhere from 0.1% to 6.8%. This translates to 16,000 patients, at the very least, who have Charcot arthropathy secondary to diabetes [2]. The ratio of men and women with Charcot arthropathy is approximately the same. It is estimated that the average duration of diabetes before onset of Charcot arthropathy is 10 years. Diabetic neuropathy has now become the leading cause of Charcot joints in the developed world [8]. Management of Charcot arthropathy of the calcaneus is less well defined than other sites in the ankle and tarsus. Unfortunately, it is no less challenging, and the principles of management in this region of the hindfoot mirror those of the other more commonly affected regions.

Pathophysiology

The pathophysiology of Charcot calcaneus includes both mechanical and physiologic factors. The Charcot foot has autonomic neuropathy of vasoregulation leading to increased blood flow and bony resorption in affected feet [9]. Not all patients demonstrate peripheral vascular disease. Impaired sensitivity combined with traumatic events regardless of magnitude are the hallmarks of this disorder. Mechanically, the neuropathic ankle offers significantly greater biomechanical challenges because of the long moment arm applied during the terminal stance phase and the poor structural quality of the host bone [10]. Charcot of the calcaneus can take different presenting forms depending on where the initial insult is sustained. The most frequent description of Charcot arthropathy is that of Eichenholtz (Table 1) [11]. It describes the spectrum of Charcot joint from the initiating incident to its final resolution. A modification has been added to Eichenholtz's original classification to include patients at risk.

Diagnosis

Charcot of the calcaneus is similar to that in other joints in that early diagnosis is imperative. The time to initial treatment is essential. Unfortunately, commonly there is a delay in recognition. The diagnosis is delayed or missed in as many as 25% of patients [12]. The clinical findings will vary depending on the stage of presentation. As noted in early stages, the swelling and skin changes can be quite striking. Distinguishing this stage from an infectious process can be challenging; however, the dependent rubor of Charcot may distinguish this from the erythema of cellulitis. Less acute stages will present with varying degrees of swelling, redness, and radiographic changes. The foot may be widened and bony prominences and ulceration may be present. Charcot arthropathy is not always painless. Patients not uncommonly will complain of pain with weight-bearing activities in addition to their neuropathic dysesthesia.

Table 1
Eichenholtz classification

Stage	Description
Stage 0, modification	Patients at risk secondary to a history of diabetes with clinical neuropathy present or diabetic patients who have sustained an acute fracture or sprain [12].
Stage I, acute dissolution phase	This is the acute inflammatory phase. It is characterized by edema, calor, erythema, and hyperemia. Radiographically, it manifests as fragmentation with dissolution and dislocation present.
Stage II, healing coalescence phase	The initial inflammatory phase has now transitioned into healing. The edema, erythema, and hyperemia begin to resolve. The radiographs exhibit new bone formation at the areas of bony destruction including the initial fracture site as well as at areas of dislocation, provided there is no major fracture present.
Stage III, resolution consolidation phase	This final phase is characterized by resolution of the destruction with healing and bony consolidation present usually with residual deformity. This phase may be difficult to identify because of the enlargement of the joint being confused with continued edema.

To assess the patient accurately, weight-bearing radiographs need to be evaluated for joint subluxation and collapse, which may not be present on standard films. Radiographs will show the typical findings of resorption, dissolution, fragmentation, dislocation, and consolidation. As expected, these findings will be somewhat stage specific. In addition, magnetic resonance imaging, bone scans, and white blood cell (WBC) scans may be used to evaluate the deformity. The WBC scan is the most specific for Charcot, but still can be questioned, especially if the patient is on antibiotics at the time of the scan. There is still difficulty in discerning Charcot from infection on most evaluations. These studies have not been shown to be conclusive. Most cases of Charcot arthropathy that do not involve ulceration are unlikely to represent cellulitis or osteomyelitis. Jirkovska and coauthors [13] found that quantitative ultrasound of the calcaneus may be a way to diagnose the acute stage of Charcot arthropathy and to assess a patient's risk of fracture. They found significant differences between the Charcot and non-Charcot foot with regard to stiffness after quantitative ultrasound of the calcaneus. The patients with acute Charcot arthropathy had significantly lower stiffness of the calcaneus in the Charcot foot than the lumbar spine and femoral neck bone mineral density. Control subjects had significantly higher calcaneal stiffness compared with the lumbar spine and femoral neck [13].

Classification

Classification of Charcot arthropathy, as with any system, is designed to suggest appropriate treatment options. Brodsky's classification describes three patterns for the Charcot foot: type 1 involves the midfoot, type 2 involves the hindfoot, and type 3A involves the ankle. Type 3B includes fracture of the calcaneus in his classification. A type 3B involves the calcaneal tuberosity. The primary problem was thought to be mechanical with joint involvement being secondary. The loss of calcaneal pitch compromises the longitudinal arch and results in Achilles insufficiency owing to shortening of the effective length of the gastrocsoleus complex [14].

Harris and Brand [15] classified 4 distinct patterns of disintegration. Pattern 1 is disintegration of the "posterior pillar," which encompasses injuries to the calcaneus. Harris believed the calcaneus in the insensate foot to be vulnerable because the foot may land more forcefully. In addition, the patient is not aware of injury, and the possibility of concurrent or previous ulceration, which may have weakened the bone via hyperemic decalcification, allows for continued deformation. Posterior pillar disintegration initiates with a fracture of the calcaneus (Fig. 1). The calcaneus deforms under continued injury and flattens. Harris and Brand [16] believed that the new stresses to the calcaneus were transverse to the trabecular alignment. The Achilles continues to pull and the calcaneus further deforms and collapses into recurvatum (Fig. 2). The tendo calcaneus loses its leverage on the foot as the recurvatum is created. The force on the anterior aspect of the foot (anterior pillar) is now changed from a horizontal to vertical force. Calcaneocuboid stabilization is lost, and this allows the talonavicular joint to subluxate dorsally [15].

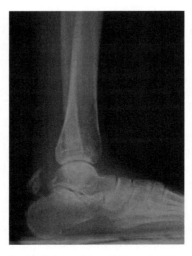

Fig. 1. Calcaneal insufficiency fracture.

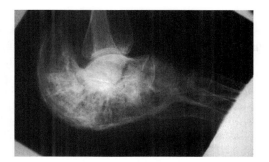

Fig. 2. Charcot calcaneal recurvatum.

The Sammarco classification scheme centers on midfoot collapse but can have inclusion of the calcaneus. Sammarco's pattern 4 is arthropathy of the first metatarsal (MT)-medial cuneiform joint with diastasis between the first and second MT. There is proximal and lateral extension into the intercuneiform joint ending at the calcaneal-cuboid joint [16].

Schon and coworkers [17] developed a four-part classification, each of which encompasses three subtypes. Type I is a lisfranc pattern, type II is the naviculocuneifrom pattern, type III the perinavicular pattern, and type IV the transverse tarsal pattern. Type IV describes calcaneal involvement.

No classification has been created that encompasses the different forces that create the different types of calcaneus lesions. The previously mentioned classifications do exhibit some limitations in their ability to fully dictate treatment. Management of a Charcot deformity of the calcaneus must incorporate knowledge of the Charcot pathophysiologic process with the biomechanical aspects of the calcaneal deformation.

Patterns of injury

Calcaneus injury occurs in three main patterns: posterior avulsion, joint depression, or anterior process fracture. Each has a different natural history. El-Khoury and Kathol [18] described four patients with avulsion fracture of the posterior tubercle of the calcaneus [19]. This finding was unusual in that the patients had no or minimal prior trauma, and all were diabetics with neuropathy. Biehl and coauthors [19] in 1993 presented cases of tuberosity fractures in neuropathic diabetics. This type of neuropathic fracture of the calcaneus has been dubbed a *calcaneal insufficiency fracture*. The Achilles spontaneously pulls off a portion of the posterior tuberosity during normal gait. Proximal migration of the tuberosity fragment may result in necrosis and possible ulceration of the overlying posterior soft tissue [20].

The second type of lesion is similar to the traumatic joint depression fractures. The difference is that this fracture is sustained with minimal trauma. It is a variant of the fracture described by Essex Lopresti [20]. The posterior facet of the subtalar joint is compressed into the body of the calcaneus.

With continued weight bearing, the talus settles into the calcaneus. The hindfoot deforms in both the sagittal and the coronal planes. Continued deformity, or deformity that leads to varus or valgus malalignment, can lead to pathologic pressure and hindfoot or ankle ulceration [20].

The third type of calcaneal injury is injury to the anterior process. An abduction force can cause compression, or an adduction force can cause avulsion of the anterior process. The fractures secondary to adduction generally cause minimal deformity. Conversely, abduction and its concomitant compression may compromise the bony integrity of the lateral column of the hindfoot. This may lead to disruption of the talonavicular joint and significant subluxation [20].

Management

The goals of treatment of Charcot arthropathy are to decrease the inflammation, encourage bone healing, and prevent further deformity [21]. Prolonged immobilization via total contact casting and bracing are used commonly to stabilize the foot in an as anatomic position as possible while reducing edema until the foot reaches the resolution phase [22]. When a patient has deformity of the foot or ankle that is severe to the point at which management with a custom brace or footwear is not feasible, or has extreme instability or persistent ulceration, operative treatment is indicated [7]. Traditionally, no operative treatment is undertaken until the arthropathy is in the Eichenholtz stage II phase. It was believed that Eichenholtz stage I inflammatory state with demineralization of the surrounding and bone as well as edema, would make operative intervention more difficult.

The first line of treatment is total contact casting. In a survey of the current practices of orthopedic surgeons, it was found that surgeons use total contact casting for 78% of their Eichenholtz stage I and 81% of their stage II patients. Interestingly, 41% and 49%, respectively, for stage I and II allowed weight bearing while being treated with total contact casting [9]. Generally, treatment of Charcot arthropathy is non–weight bearing. This treatment is often prolonged as it may take up to 18 months for fracture healing [2]. Some investigators believe that allowing weight bearing too soon can result in continued displacement and fragmentation, which can lead to loss of bony structure. Biehl and coauthors [19] treated avulsion fractures of the calcaneal tuberosity with a serial short leg non–weight bearing casts with the foot positioned in equinus for several months. Schon and coauthors [6] also treated posterior calcaneal tuberosity avulsions with casting with good results. Casting can also be used to attempt to heal ulceration before surgical intervention.

Surgical intervention on the neuropathic foot must be judicious. In general terms, surgery may encompass debridement with or without exostectomy or exostectomy alone, or it may involve arthrodesis. Select fractures, such as tuberosity avulsion, may require operative fixation to preserve the soft tissue envelope. As with any operative intervention, meticulous soft tissue handling is paramount. Indications must include an assessment of the patient's function, vascular supply, and comorbidities. As always, compliance must be addressed when managing these complex situations.

Debridement and exostectomy

Surgical treatment with ulcers present has been attempted with dismal results. Thompson and Clohisy performed surgery on patients with open plantar ulcerations. These procedures resulted in a 25% incidence of deep infections. This is compared with a zero incidence of deep infections when the procedure was performed on a patient with intact skin [15]. As the deformities of the calcaneus increase, total contact casting becomes less of a viable option.

Farber and coauthors [8] realized the difficulty in healing some ulceration with total contact casting. They treated 11 patients with Charcot and midfoot collapse with ulceration. They performed a corrective osteotomy with surgical debridement. The patient was placed in an external fixator for postoperative stabilization rather than a total contact cast. None of their patients had a recurrence of their ulcers. At the conclusion of the study, all patients were able to wear custom shoe wear, and 10 of the 11 were able to ambulate to perform activities of daily living. Prokuski and Saltzman [21] treated bilateral Charcot of the ankle in external fixators with good results. They found that skin breakdown from casting was eliminated, and the fixators provided excellent stabilization of the neuropathic joint. They advocated for close follow-up owing to the possibility of pin tract infections and the need for prolonged non–weight bearing.

Another option to address the difficulty of healing of calcaneal ulcerations is partial excision of the os calcis. Brodsky and Rouse [23] performed successful exostectomies for Brodsky type I (midfoot) and II (hindfoot not specifically calcaneus) Charcot arthropathy. However, there was a 25% rate of complications that was related directly to soft tissue healing. The patient in his study with the worst outcome had the worst soft tissues initially. He believed that the surgeon must achieve a balance between resection enough to prevent continual ulceration and resecting too much and causing further instability. Smith and coworkers [24] specifically addressed exostectomy of the calcaneus. They performed partial excision of os calcis on neuropathic patients with ulceration of os calcis. Of the 10 patients, four healed in 26 weeks, three still had open areas but were functional, and three progressed to amputation. This represents a 70% functional success rate, but only 40% surgical success.

Bollinger and Thordarson [25] reported their experience with calcanectomy as a salvage to below-knee amputation. Their results supported the role for partial calcanectomy in individuals with chronic heel ulcers with or without osteomyelitis. Advantages include the ability to use a shoe with a modified insert, avoiding the increased energy expenditure experienced with below knee amputation.

Arthrodesis

When total contact casting, debridement, and exostectomy fail, the surgeon must consider arthrodesis. Arthrodesis historically has been considered a salvage procedure. Thompson and Clohisy [26] looked at deformity owing to Charcot arthropathy in the region of the ankle or tarsal bones. Each of the five extremities that had deformity in the region of the ankle and hindfoot had substantial loss of bone that resulted in instability and severe malalignment. They found that the frequency of failed attempts at reconstruction of neuropathic joins of the foot or ankle was approximately 60%. Their study indicated that factors that play a role in a failed reconstruction are infection and previous failed reconstruction. Patients who do not have ulcers but cannot be managed with the use of a load-sharing device could benefit from operative reconstruction. However, patients who have persistent deformity-related ulcers should await ulcer healing before having a major surgical reconstruction.

Common contraindications to arthrodesis surgery include (1) Eichenholtz stage I Charcot joint, (2) malnutrition or uncontrolled diabetes, (3) soft tissue infection, (4) peripheral vascular disease, (5) poor bone quality unable to hold fixation, and (6) known poor patient compliance with postoperative directives such as weight bearing status and bracing. Despite these contraindications, arthrodesis often is undertaken in less-than-ideal patients. This stems from the fact that the only other option is amputation. In addition to the fact that most diabetics are at risk for the possibility of contralateral involvement, the cost of reconstruction has been noted to be less than amputation. Cost of a reconstruction group during a 5-year period was 14% less than the total cost of a below-knee amputation group for the same period [16].

The principles of fusion of a Charcot joint stem from the work of Drennan and colleagues [27] regarding arthrodesis of the knee [28]. They asserted that a successful fusion of a Charcot joint required removal of all cartilage, debris, and sclerotic bone. Included in this debridement was resection of all synovial and scarred capsular tissue. The bone surfaces needed to be down to vascularized bleeding bone with reduction maximizing bony surface [28]. Bono and coauthors [29] examined arthrodesis of the subtalar, ankle, and pantalar joints. Using arthrodesis as a salvage procedure after failure of nonoperative treatment, they achieved 91% clinical union and stability. Early and Hansen [22] treated nine patients with Brodsky type II Charcot arthropathy. All the patients underwent subtalar complex stabilization and fusion of midtarsal structures. They achieved limb salvage in seven of the nine feet. The time to union was 5 months. Of the two failed treatments, one patient went on to below-knee amputation, and the other died in the early postoperative period. Papa and coauthors [30] found clinical stability in 93% of their patients who underwent arthrodesis of various joints as a salvage procedure for Charcot joints. This was despite a 31% pseudoarthrosis rate.

The previous arthrodeses were accomplished with either interfragmentary screws, staples, or Steinman pins. Pinzur and Kelikian [10] advocated arthrodesis of the subtalar joint using a retrograde intramedullary rodding technique. They performed retrograde nailing of the subtalar joint through the calcaneus and talus (if possible) and into the tibia of 21 ankles. Nineteen of the 21 ankles fused at an average of 20 months of follow-up. Patients who were able to retain their talus had clinical and radiographic fusion at an average of 5.3 months. Ten of 21 patients with poor calcaneal quality either required resection of the talus or had deformity of the talus that required resection and had their intramedullary rod rotated 90° to facilitate locking screws in a posterior to anterior projection. In this subset of patients, Pinzur and Kelikian advised that due consideration should be given also to the possibility of ankle disarticulation as their healing was prolonged [10]. Chi and coauthors [31] found that the use of a lateral one third tubular plate as a buttress worked well in patients whose bone was too soft to use standard locking bolts and washers for intramedullary rod fixation or in the case of fusion revisions.

Even when successful arthrodesis is achieved, there persists the potential for morbidity. A long-moment arm is created when both the tibiotalar and subtalar joint are arthrodesed. The body must clear this extended lever arm with each step. This creates new stress at the ends of the arthrodesis. Mitchell and coworkers [32] reported on tibial stress fractures secondary to fusion in neuropathic patients. Of note, two of the three patients who sustained the stress fractures were not compliant with their prescription footwear or brace wear. Tibial stress fracture should be discussed as a possible complication of arthrodesis surgery in the Charcot patient.

Thus far, all arthrodesis procedures had been performed in patients who were Eichenholtz phase II. This unfortunately allowed the patients in phase I to continue to experience collapse and fragment if their deformities could not be contained. Simon and colleagues [33] performed arthrodesis in Eichenholtz stage I. All arthrodesis were successful. They had anatomic reduction, clinical union, and stability without any increased risk of complications. Before this study, the common thought was that operative intervention should not occur while the patient was still in stage I because it would lead to poor outcomes and further fragmentation and bony destruction.

Summary

Charcot of the calcaneus, although not as prolific as midfoot deformation, still results in significant morbidity. Current treatment centers on methods proven effective for other joints in the foot. Most neuropathic conditions of the calcaneus can be managed reasonably nonoperatively. In cases of severe deformity or ulceration, surgical management may be the more conservative approach. The surgical principles of proper soft tissue balancing and handling are critical. As the diabetic population continues to increase, the incidence of Charcot of the calcaneus will concomitantly increase. Further research into methods of arthrodesis and osteotomy with external fixation seem to be the direction of the future.

References

[1] Charcot J. Lectures on the diseases of the nervous system. Sigerson G, translator. London: The New Sydenham Society; 1868.
[2] Esses S, Langer F, Gross A. Charcot's joints: a case report in a young patient with diabetes. Clin Orthop 1981;156:183–6.
[3] Gupta R. A short history of neuropathic arthropathy. Clin Orthop 1993;296:43–9.
[4] Bailey C, Root HE. Neuropathic joint lesions in diabetes mellitus. J Clin Invest 1942;21:649.
[5] Coventry M, Rothacker G. Bilateral calcaneal fracture in a diabetic patient. J Bone Joint Surg 1979;61A(3):462–4.
[6] Schon L, Easley M, Weinfeld S. Charcot neuropathy of the foot and ankle. Clin Orthop 1998;349:116–31.
[7] Johnson J. Operative treatment of neuropathic arthropathy of the foot and ankle. J Bone Joint Surg 1998;80A(11):1700–9.
[8] Farber D, Juliano P, Cavanagh P, et al. Single stage correction with external fixation of the ulcerated foot in individuals with Charcot neuropathy. Foot Ankle Int 2002;23(2):130–4.
[9] Pinzur M, Shields N, Trepman E, et al. Current practice patterns in the treatment of Charcot foot. Foot Ankle Int 2000;21(11):916–20.
[10] Pinzur M, Kelikian A. Charcot ankle fusion with a retrograde locked intramedullary nail. Foot Ankle Int 1997;18(11):699–703.
[11] Eichenholtz S. Charcot joints. Springfield (IL): Charles C. Thomas; 1966.
[12] Marks R. Complications of foot and ankle surgery in patients with diabetes. Clin Orthop 2001;391:153–61.
[13] Jirkovska A, Kasalicky P, Boucetk P, et al. Calcaneal ultrasonometry in patients with Charcot osteoarthropathy and its relationship with densitometry in the lumbar spine and femoral neck and with markers of bone turnover. Diabet Med 2001;18:495–500.
[14] Graves M, Tarquino T. Diabetic neuropathy (Charcot joints): the importance of recognizing chronic sensory deficits in the treatment of acute foot and ankle fractures in diabetic patients. Orthopedics 2003;26(4):415–8.
[15] Harris J, Brand P. Patterns of disintegration of the tarsus in the anaesthetic foot. J Bone Joint Surg 1966;48B(1):4–16.
[16] Sammarco G, Conti S. Surgical treatment of neuropathic foot deformity. Foot Ankle Int 1998;19(2):102–9.
[17] Schon LC, Easley ME, Weonfeld SB. Charcot neuroarthropathy of the foot and ankle. Clin Orthop 1998;359:116–31.
[18] El-Khoury GY, Kathol MH. Neuropathic fractures in patients with diabetes mellitus. Radiology 1982;144:137.
[19] Biehl W, Morgan J, Wagner W, et al. Neuropathic calcaneal tuberosity avulsion fractures. Clin Orthop 1993;296:8–13.
[20] Campbell J. Intra-articular neuropathic fracture of the calcaneal body treated by open reduction and subtalar arthrodesis. Foot Ankle Int 2001;22(5):440–4.
[21] Prokuski L, Saltzman C. External fixation for the treatment of Charcot arthropathy of the ankle: a case report. Foot Ankle Int 1998;19(5):336–41.
[22] Early J, Hansen S. Surgical reconstruction of the diabetic foot: a salvage approach for midfoot collapse. Foot Ankle Int 1996;17(6):325–30.

[23] Brodsky J, Rouse A. Exostectomy for symptomatic bony prominences in diabetic Charcot feet. Clin Orthop 1993;296:21–6.
[24] Smith W, Jacobs R, Fuchs M. Salvage of the diabetic foot with exposed os calcis. Clin Orthop 1993;296:71–7.
[25] Bollinger M, Thordarson DB. Partial calcanectomy: an alternative to below knee amputation. Foot Ankle Int 2002;23(10):927–32.
[26] Thompson R, Clohisy D. Deformity following fracture in diabetic neuropathic osteoarthropathy. J Bone Joint Surg 1993;75(12):1765–73.
[27] Drennan DB, Fahey JJ, Maylan DJ. Important factors in achieving arthrodesis of the Charcot knee. J Bone Joint Surg 1971;53A:1180–93.
[28] Alvarez R, Barbour T, Perkins T. Tibiocalcaneal Arthodesis for nonbraceable neuropathic ankle deformity. Foot Ankle Int 1994;15(7):354–9.
[29] Bono J, Roger D, Jacobs R. Surgical arthrodesis of the neuropathic foot. Clin Orthop 1993; 296:14–20.
[30] Papa J, Myerson M, Girard P. Salvage, with arthrodesis, in intractable diabetic neuropathic arthropathy of the foot and ankle. J Bone Joint Surg 1993;75A(7):1056–66.
[31] Chi T, McWilliam J, Gould J. Lateral plate-washer technique for revision tibiocalcaneal fusion. Am J Orthop 2001;30(7):588–90.
[32] Mitchell J, Johnson J, Collier B, et al. Stress fracture of the tibia following extensive hindfoot ankle arthrodesis: a report of three cases. Foot & Ank Int 1995;16(7):445–8.
[33] Simon S, Tejwani S, Wilson D, et al. Arthrodesis as an early alternative to nonoperative management of Charcot arthropathy of the diabetic foot. J Bone Joint Surg 2000;82A(7): 939–50.

ELSEVIER
SAUNDERS

Foot Ankle Clin N Am
11 (2006) 837–847

FOOT AND
ANKLE CLINICS

The Role of Ring External Fixation in Charcot Foot Arthropathy

Michael S. Pinzur, MD

Loyola University Medical Center, 2160 South First Avenue, Maywood, IL 60153, USA

Diabetes-associated Charcot arthropathy of the foot and ankle imparts a severe negative impact on the health-related quality of life of affected individuals [1–3]. The treatment of affected patients is very controversial. Although most orthopedic textbooks advise accommodative care with orthotic devices, most peer-reviewed publications offer retrospective level IV evidence that surgical correction is the preferred method of treatment. This controversy can be understood better if one defines what is meant by a favorable outcome. If simple limb preservation and limited walking capacity is the desired goal, then accommodative methods with a CROW (Charcot restraint orthotic walker) or ankle-foot orthotic variant generally can be successful [4–6]. If a favorable outcome is defined as an ambulatory patient who is ulcer free and is capable of being managed long-term with commercially available therapeutic footwear (ie, commercially available depth-inlay shoes and custom accommodative foot orthoses), then resection of the infected bone and surgical correction of the deformity is necessary.

A therapeutic algorithm has evolved that suggests that as many as 60% of these patients can be treated successfully without surgery [7,8]. Patients who are determined to be clinically plantigrade at the time of presentation and have a reasonably colinear talar–first metatarsal axis (as determined by weight-bearing anterior–posterior radiographs), will likely achieve the desired favorable outcome after treatment with a weight-bearing total contact cast (Fig. 1) [9].

Surgical candidates

Patients are considered nonplantigrade when they are bearing weight on tissue that is not capable of absorbing the pressure and shear forces associated with weight bearing. These deformities can be severe varus or valgus of

E-mail address: mpinzu1@lumc.edu

1083-7515/06/$ - see front matter © 2006 Elsevier Inc. All rights reserved.
doi:10.1016/j.fcl.2006.06.006

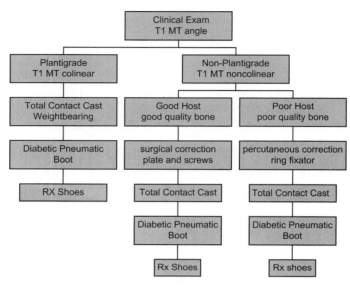

Fig. 1. Therapeutic algorithm for treatment of Charcot foot osteoarthropathy. Patients who are clinically plantigrade and have a collinear talar–first metatarsal axis determined from weight-bearing radiographs, are treated with a total contact cast, and progress to a pneumatic boot, and eventually to therapeutic footwear. Those patients deemed to be nonplantigrade, are treated with surgery, followed by a total contact cast, pneumatic boot, and therapeutic footwear.

the forefoot as compared with the hindfoot. Those designated as non-plantigrade will generally have a common nonplantigrade deformity that is not capable of being accommodated is the classic severe "rocker-bottom" deformity. Patients who are considered likely to have ulceration over a bony deformity can be identified both clinically and radiographically. Those designated as nonplantigrade, will have a noncolinear talar–first metatarsal axis, as determined from weight-bearing radiographs (Fig. 2). These patients may achieve early resolution of the destructive neuropathic arthropathy process with a total contact cast but are at risk for the late development of full-thickness ulcers and contiguous osteomyelitis, if their deformity is not corrected (Fig. 3) [10–15]. These patients pose unique challenges. They generally are morbidly obese [16]. The bone in the region of the neuropathic arthropathy is often osteopenic, making surgical correction and maintenance of that reduction difficult [17]. These patients are complicated further by poor white blood cell function, impaired immunity, and an increased risk of surgically acquired infection [18].

Treatment strategy

An ideal method for correction of these severe deformities would involve minimal surgical dissection and a method of maintaining the corrected

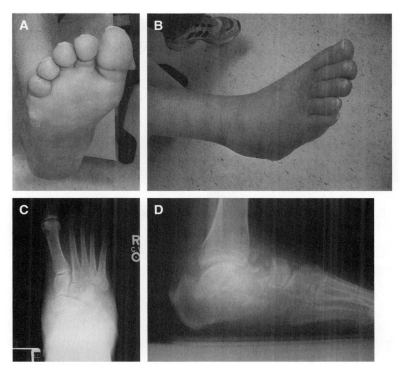

Fig. 2. (*A, B*) This patient was clinically plantigrade at the time of presentation. (*C, D*) Weight-bearing radiographs show a collinear talar–first metatarsal axis on the anterior-posterior view. He was allowed to weight bear in a total contact cast that was changed every 2 weeks until the foot stabilized. He progressed to commercially available therapeutic footwear (depth-inlay shoes and custom accommodative foot orthoses). He has remained ambulatory, active, and ulcer-free for several years.

alignment while allowing the patient to bear weight. Standard methods of internal fixation are dependent on the pullout strength of screws, or a plate and screw construct. The principles of Illizarov appear to be ideally suited for this complex patient population. This method allows minimal surgical dissection and exposure to simply correct the deformity. Through a small incision, a predetermined wedge of bone can be resected that will allow correction of the multiple plane deformity. Extended surgical dissection to place large implants is not necessary. The use of fine wire ring fixation minimizes the risk for mechanical failure in poor quality bone. The down side to this option is the inherent fear that most orthopedic surgeons possess when considering using fine wire ring external fixation for the dynamic correction of deformity.

Use of the ring fixator as a dynamic method of achieving correction of deformity is the process that dissuades most practicing orthopedic surgeons from using ring external fixation. The technique conjures up thoughts

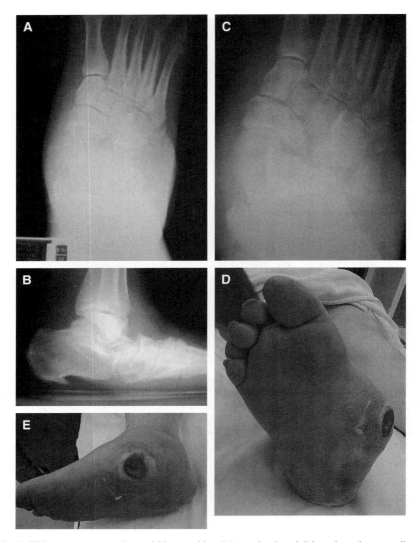

Fig. 3. This woman currently would be considered "nonplantigrade" based on the noncolinear talar–first metatarsal axis, measured from a weight-bearing radiograph. She had no skin breakdown at her initial presentation (*A, B*), or at 1 year (*C*). She returned for follow-up every 2 months. Two years later, in spite of wearing therapeutic footwear, this skin breakdown developed (*D, E*), which eventually led to transtibial amputation.

derived during residency of prolonged surgical times, and the complications related to limb lengthening, and the gradual correction of the deformity. The external fixation frames are complex to build and require daily maintenance. This strategy involves percutaneous or open correction of bony deformity, a concept that is well within the domain of the practicing

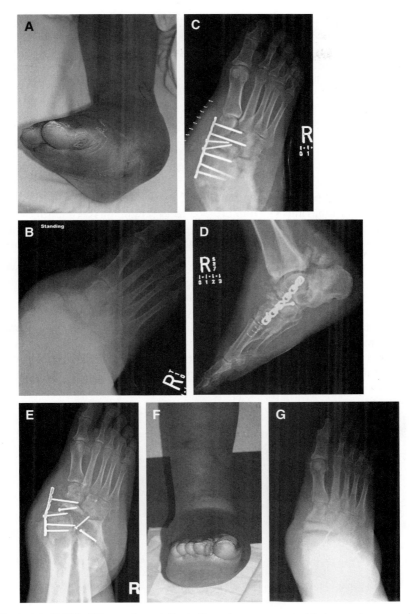

Fig. 4. (*A, B*) This 400-pound mentally challenged man was not able to remain non–weight bearing. He tried to remain non–weight bearing after correction of his deformity (*C, D*), and this recurrent deformity developed 2 months later (*E*). He was successfully revised with percutaneous correction and application of a ring fixator (*F, G*).

orthopedic surgeon. Once the deformity is corrected, a simplified, preassembled, nonadjustable version of a ring fixator can be used simply to maintain the correction achieved at surgery. Surgery time can be minimized with this technique by pre-assembling the neutral external fixation frame (Figs. 4 and 5).

Patient selection

The first step in the decision-making process is to determine which 60% of the patients can be treated without surgery [4,7–9]. The next step is distinguishing relatively low-risk surgical candidates from high-risk candidates. Low-risk surgical patients can be managed by any of a number of methods of internal fixation, ranging from crossed large fragment screws, long intramedullary screws, or plate and screw fixation constructs [8,10–14]. Assigning a patient to a high-risk status is arbitrary and is based on several factors:

- The most obvious risk factor is the presence of osteomyelitis with a draining overlying wound. In the past, it has been recommended anecdotally to perform a preliminary debridement of the infection and treat with culture-specific antibiotic therapy. The definitive surgery then is delayed until the wound heals. Although reasonably safe, this process may take months or years to achieve wound healing in a patient who is required to be non–weight bearing during this period. Placing a foreign body at the time of debridement carries a high risk for foreign body–associated osteomyelitis.

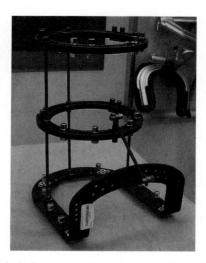

Fig. 5. Nonadjustable prebuilt frame generally used to maintain surgically acquired correction. (Depuy, Inc., Warsaw, Indiana).

- Morbid obesity makes both achieving and maintaining stability difficult. In addition, it is virtually impossible for such patients to maintain a non–weight-bearing, or limited weight-bearing status.
- Localized osteopenia may be caused by disuse during a prolonged period of treatment and limited weight bearing, or may be caused by the pathophysiology of the disease process. Patients with poor quality bone are more likely to have mechanical complications.
- Many longstanding diabetics also have an impaired immune system. These individuals will have impaired white blood cell function as well as impaired T-cell immunity.

Surgical technique

A morbidly obese (350+ pounds) diabetic female patient with a complicated deformity shows the steps in achieving correction of the multiple plane deformity and stabilization with a simple prebuilt ring external fixator. This patient was treated initially with a total contact cast and treated for several years with custom fabricated therapeutic footwear. She was referred for treatment after stumbling and developing new-onset swelling of the foot. Progressive deformity developed while she was being treated with a total contact cast (Fig. 6).

The first step at surgery was an Achilles tendon lengthening or gastrocnemius lengthening to achieve motor balance from the deforming motor peripheral neuropathy. Applying the principles of Illizarov, a small incision was used to perform a corrective osteotomy with a power saw. A predetermined wedge of bone was removed to allow correction of the deformity. A pre-assembled ring external fixation frame (see Fig. 5) was slid over the foot. The first step was to position the foot safely below the lowest ring and avoiding any localized contact with the ring. Thirty-degree olive wires were placed in the calcaneus. These olive wires were attached to the distal ring and tensioned with an external tensioning device. With the foot held in the corrected position, 30° olive wires were placed through the metatarsals, and the forefoot was secured to the circular frame with tensioned olive wires. The ankle was positioned at neutral, and the two proximal circular rings were secured to the tibia with obliquely placed tensioned olive wires.

Treatment examples

A 400-pound, 37-year-old mentally challenged man worked in a sheltered workshop. The patient had several partial-thickness ulcers over the head of his talus in spite of the use of custom therapeutic footwear. He was not capable of ambulating without bearing weight on this foot. Initially he underwent tendon Achilles lengthening and surgical correction of the deformity, using a hybrid system of internal fixation. He was treated postoperatively

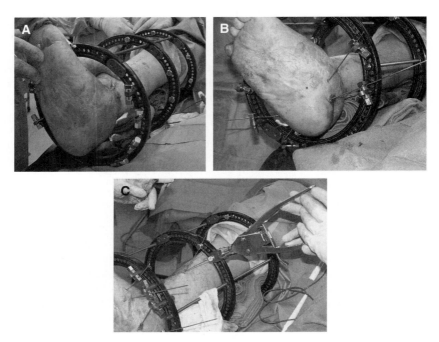

Fig. 6. Surgical technique. (*A*) After correction of the deformity, the pre-assembled frame is slipped over the foot. (*B*) Taking care to have the foot free from contact with the frame, olive wires are placed through the heel at a 30° angle and then tensioned. (*C*) The forefoot is then positioned. Olive wires are placed at 30° through the metatarsal shafts and tensioned. Wires then are tensioned at two levels in the tibia, and tensioned, being careful to have no direct contact to the frame.

in a total contact cast and was asked to attempt to limit his weight bearing. He appeared to be progressing to union 6 weeks after surgery. At 8 weeks, although still protected with a total contact cast, it was apparent that the fixation had failed. Most of the hardware was removed through the initial surgical incision. The osteotomy site was "freshened." The deformity was corrected again, achieving a plantigrade foot. A "jumbo" frame with 10-inch rings was used for 8 weeks during which the patient attempted to limit his weight bearing. A weight bearing total contact cast then was used for an additional 4 weeks, when the patient was transitioned to commercially available therapeutic footwear (Fig. 4).

This second example illustrates the ability to apply the principles of Illizarov to this simplified technique using the ring external fixator simply as the conduit to maintain a surgically achieved correction of deformity. This patient had renal failure and purulent drainage from the posterior ankle. The ankle was debrided, and culture-specific antibiotic therapy was initiated. The ring external fixator was used to allow bony healing (Fig. 7).

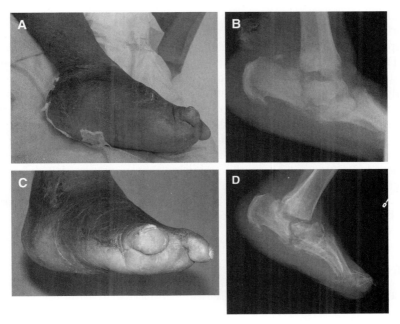

Fig. 7. (*A, B*) This renal failure patient had purulent drainage from this infected Charcot foot. (*C*) The infection was debrided, and the patient was treated with culture-specific parenteral antibiotic therapy. (*D*) At 1 year, she has a stable foot with no recurrence of the infection.

Summary

These two morbidly obese patients with severe Charcot foot arthropathy were treated successfully with percutaneous correction of their deformity followed by a stepwise application of a pre-assembled neutrally aligned multiplane ring external fixator. This technique transfers well to the trauma environment in which alignment can be maintained without further violation within the zone of injury.

The application of fine wire ring external fixation has been used for many years to accomplish leg lengthening and correction of deformity. Historically, it has required a great deal of experience to apply the complex frames and implement the required daily adjustments. The patient experience often has been an unpleasant ordeal with a high potential for associated morbidity. This negative exposure has prompted practicing orthopedic surgeons to avoid this technique, feeling that it best be left to those in a tertiary care setting who are equipped to handle the morbidity and complications.

Taking this technology from the domain of the deformity surgeon to the general orthopedic community will require the suppression of bad memories from residency. Using the device solely as a method of maintaining alignment eliminates many of the dynamic attributes that contribute to pain and morbidity. The bone and soft tissues are not stretched, eliminating much of the pain and decreasing the rate of traction-associated pin tract morbidity. Because there is no dynamic component of the treatment, the simplified frame can be pre-assembled and have no adjustable components.

The experience derived from this application has the potential of expanding the role of ring external fixation. Where the frame has been used previously as method of both obtaining and maintaining alignment, this application uses a simplified neutral version of a complex device to simply maintain alignment in a high-risk patient population. Correction of deformity and achieving alignment/reduction of fractures is well within the domain of the practicing orthopedic surgeon. Once that correction has been achieved, this application simply maintains that correction. It helps avoid extensive surgical dissection in a poor host and eliminates the need for bone that is mechanically capable of holding internal fixation devices during the bony and soft tissue healing period.

References

[1] Pinzur MS, Evans A. Health related quality of life in patients with Charcot foot. Am J Ortho 2003;32:492–6.
[2] Dhawan V, Spratt KF, Pinzur MS, et al. Reliability of AOFAS Diabetic Foot Questionnaire in Charcot arthropathy: stability, internal consistency and measurable difference. Foot Ank Int 2005;26:717–31.
[3] Saltzman CL, Domsic RT, Baumhauer JF, et al. Foot and ankle research priority: report from the Research Council of the American Orthopaedic Foot and Ankle Society. Foot Ankle Int 1997;18:443–6.
[4] Pinzur MS, Dart H. Pedorthic management of the diabetic foot. Foot Ankle Clin 2001;6: 205–14.
[5] Brodsky JW. The diabetic foot. In: Coughlin MJ, Mann RA, editors. Surgery of the foot and ankle. 7th edition. St. Louis (MO): Mosby; 1999. p. 895–969.
[6] Morgan JM, Biehl WC III, Wagner FWW Jr. Management of neuropathic arthropathy with the charcot restraint orthotic walker. Clin Orthop 1993;296:58–63.
[7] Pinzur MS. Surgical vs. accommodative treatment for charcot arthropathy of the midfoot. Foot Ank Int 2004;25:545–9.
[8] Pinzur MS, Sage R, Stuck R, et al. A treatment algorithm for neuropathic (charcot) midfoot deformity. Foot Ankle Int 1993;14:189–97.
[9] Bevan WP, Tomlinson MP. Radiographic measure as a predictor of ulcer formation in midfoot charcot. Presented at the Annual Meeting of the American Orthopaedic Foot and Ankle Society. www.aofas.org. Seattle, July, 2004.
[10] Alpert SW, Koval KJ, Zuckerman JD. Neuropathic arthropathy: review of current knowledge. J Am Acad Orthop Surg 1996;4:100–8.
[11] Early JS, Hansen ST. Surgical reconstruction of the diabetic foot. Foot Ankle Int 1996;17: 325–30.
[12] Myerson MS, Henderson MR, Saxby T, et al. Management of midfoot diabetic neuroarthropathy. Foot Ankle Int 1994;15:233–41.
[13] Papa J, Myerson M, Girard P. Salvage, with arthrodesis, in intractable diabetic neuropathic arthropathy of the foot and ankle. J Bone Joint Surg 1993;75A:1056–66.
[14] Simon SR, Tejwani SG, Wilson DL, et al. Arthrodesis as an early alternative to nonoperative management of charcot arthropathy of the diabetic foot. J Bone Joint Surg 2000;82A: 939–50.

[15] Farber DC, Juliano PJ, Cavanagh PR, et al. Single stage correction with external fixation of the ulcerated foot in individuals with charcot neuroarthropathy. Foot Ank Int 2002;23: 130–4.

[16] Pinzur MS, Freeland R, Juknelis D. The association between body mass index and diabetic foot disorders. Foot Ank Int 2005;26:375–7.

[17] Herbst SA, Jones KB, Saltzman CL. Pattern of diabetic neuropathic arthropathy associated with the peripheral bone mineral density. J Bone Joint Surg 2004;86B:378–83.

[18] Bibbo C, Lin SS, Beam HA, et al. Complications of ankle fractures in diabetic patients. Ortho Clin North Am 2001;32:113–33.

ELSEVIER
SAUNDERS

Foot Ankle Clin N Am
11 (2006) 849–863

FOOT AND
ANKLE CLINICS

Ankle Fractures in Diabetics

Victor R. Prisk, MD, Dane K. Wukich, MD*

*Department of Orthopaedic Surgery, University of Pittsburgh, 3471 Fifth Avenue,
Kaufman Building Suite 1010, Pittsburgh, PA 15213, USA*

Diabetes mellitus affects millions of people and has a continually increasing prevalence in the United States population [1]. The American diabetic population has more than doubled from 5.8 million to 13.8 million between 1980 and 2003. Between 1996 and 1997, there was a great increase in the number of Americans with diabetes diagnosed, likely owing to changes in diagnostic criteria [1,2]. The Centers for Disease Control and Prevention estimate that more than 5 million Americans have undiagnosed diabetes mellitus. The number of new cases of diabetes has increased by 52% from 1997 through 2003. Approximately 17% of persons with diabetes fall between the ages of 65 and 74 years.

In addition to having diabetes and its associated medical conditions, diabetics often have other risk factors for medical complications. Eighteen percent of adults in the United States who have diabetes smoke tobacco, 37% are sedentary, 82% are overweight, and up to 60% have other cardiovascular risk factors [1].

Diabetes mellitus is a group of metabolic disorders with the common manifestation of hyperglycemia. This hyperglycemia results in the nonenzymatic glycosylation of proteins and increased formation of intracellular sorbitol and other polyols that causes tissue damage in almost all organ systems. This results in immune dysfunction, peripheral neuropathy, macro- and micro-angiopathy, nephropathy, retinopathy, and neuropathic arthropathy.

Each year approximately 260,000 Americans sustain an ankle fracture [3], and approximately 25% patients with these fractures undergo surgical stabilization. The rate of surgical stabilization for isolated lateral malleolus fractures has been approximately 10%, and increases to 20% for isolated medial malleolus fractures, almost 60% for bimalleolar fractures, and 70% for trimalleolar fractures [4]. Ganesh and coauthors [5] studied

---

* Corresponding author.
E-mail address: wukichdk@upmc.edu (D.K. Wukich).

1083-7515/06/$ - see front matter © 2006 Elsevier Inc. All rights reserved.
doi:10.1016/j.fcl.2006.06.013
foot.theclinics.com

160,598 patients with ankle fractures and found that nearly 6% of those patients had diabetes mellitus. There have been several studies focusing on the unique features of the treatment of ankle fractures in diabetics. In this report, the challenges presented by treating the diabetic with an ankle fracture are reviewed.

Diabetic comorbidities

Neuropathy

Of the more than 18 million diabetic patients in the United States, up to 40% have peripheral neuropathy within the first decade of diabetes onset [6,7]. Ten percent of all diabetics have some form of neuropathy at the time of diagnosis. Retinopathy, nephropathy, and peripheral vascular disease are often present concomitantly with neuropathy. More than 50% of diabetics greater than 60 years old have some degree of peripheral neuropathy [8]. Peripheral neuropathy can manifest as abnormalities in sensory, motor, or autonomic function. Hyperglycemia leads to increased activity in the polyol pathway in nerve cells, resulting in abnormal nerve function through osmotic stress [9]. Abnormal vibratory sensation and decreased gastrosoleus reflex have been noted in approximately 90% of diabetics with neuropathy [6]. Autonomic dysfunction may be present and manifests as dry cracking skin and alterations in cutaneous perfusion. Motor dysfunction may manifest as contractures of the intrinsic muscles of the foot causing clawing of the toes.

Peripheral neuropathy is usually profound before leading to loss of protective sensation. Protective sensation is the threshold of sensation below which the patient has a measurably increased risk of diabetic foot ulceration [10]. Once protective sensation is lost, a seven-fold increased risk in foot ulceration occurs because of vulnerability to physical and thermal trauma [11,12]. Although the "gold standard" for diagnosing peripheral neuropathy is nerve conduction studies, the most frequently used instrument for the detection of protective sensation is the 10 g/5.07 nylon Semmes-Weinstein monofilament [13]. The Semmes-Weinstein monofilament can identify persons at increased risk of foot ulceration with a sensitivity of up to 91%, and a specificity of up to 86% [14–16]. Ninety percent of patients with an insensate location can be identified by testing just four plantar sites on the forefoot (great toe and the first, third, and fifth metatarsals) [17]. Some consider a lack of perception at any site to be abnormal. As the threshold for an abnormal test is increased from one to four insensate sites, the sensitivity remains greater than 90%, whereas the specificity improves from 60% to 80% [18]. Use of a tuning fork for vibratory sense is less predictive of ulceration than monofilament testing [14]. A case–control study testing 255 diabetic persons found that either abnormal Semmes-Weinstein monofilament perception or a vibration–perception threshold of more than 25V via a biothesiometer is predictive of foot ulceration with a sensitivity of 100% and a specificity of 77% [19].

Arthropathy

Peripheral neuropathy may lead to many of the complications that occur with ankle fractures in diabetics. In particular, peripheral neuropathy appears to be essential in the development of Charcot neuroarthropathy [20]. Loss of sensibility in the diabetic patient results in a reduction in pain, thermal sensation, loss of light touch, and proprioception [21]. This reduction in sensation results in an inability to sense minor traumatic events, whether it be a new trauma or unknowingly applying too much weight to an injured or at-risk limb. It is theorized that normal muscle reflexes are reduced resulting in progressive eccentric loading and joint deformity [22]. Animal studies and clinical observations have found that appropriate immobilization of an injured extremity in those with peripheral neuropathy can limit the rapidly progressive cartilage destruction and joint deformity of Charcot neuroarthropathy [23–24]. The autonomic dysfunction seen with peripheral neuropathy in diabetics may also contribute to the arthropathy and the observed osteopenia caused by increased blood flow and abnormal osteoclastic activity [20].

Angiopathy

Diabetes is present in up to 41% of patients with peripheral arterial disease [25]. Costigan and Thordarson [26] have reported that peripheral neuropathy and peripheral vascular disease are significant factors in the complication rate after operative management of ankle fractures in diabetics. Diabetics have both micro- and macro-angiopathies that develop progressively. The atherosclerotic disease, most often affecting the popliteal trifurcation and sparing pedal vessels [27], may result in diminished blood flow and diminished or absent pulses, and thus a reduction in nutrient supply to the peripheral tissues. Diabetics are prone to intrinsic wound-healing disturbances, such as impaired collagen cross-linking and matrix metalloproteinase function, decreased granulocyte function, and malnutrition, all of which lead to an increased risk of infection [27–30].

All diabetics with ankle fractures should be examined closely for peripheral vascular disease. This begins with the examination of the dorsalis pedis and posterior tibial pulses. If pulses are found to be diminished or absent, then a noninvasive vascular examination is critical. Peripheral vascular disease is detected most easily by the ankle-brachial index (ABI), which is the ratio of systolic blood pressure in the ankle to that in the brachial artery. An ABI ratio of 0.90 or less suggests peripheral vascular disease [27]. However, an ABI of 1.1 or higher may represent a falsely elevated pressure caused by medial arterial calcinosis, making the vessel less compressible by the pressure cuff [27]. If the ABI result suggests peripheral vascular disease, pre-operative vascular consultation is recommended.

Transcutaneous oxygen measurements are useful in patients with ankle fracture, because these patients may not tolerate a blood pressure cuff around their injured ankle. A transcutaneous oxygen pressure (T_cPo_2) higher than 30 mm Hg correlates with a high likelihood of wound healing [27]. A T_cPo_2 less than 30 mm Hg indicates limb ischemia and necessitates a vascular consultation with angiography or possibly a revascularization procedure [31,32]. Bongard and Krahenbuhl suggested that a 10–mm Hg increase in T_cPo_2 on inhaled oxygen may be a better predictor of potential wound healing than static T_cPo_2 measurements in the diabetic [33]. The reported effect of revascularization procedures on the incidence and site of amputations varies, but most recent findings suggest benefits [34,35].

Delayed fracture healing

In general, patients with both types I and II diabetes take nearly twice as long to heal displaced lower extremity fractures and fractures treated by open reduction [36]. Sinacore [37] found that acute Charcot neuropathic arthropathies with fracture, subluxation, or dislocation healed, on average, in 86 days. Additionally, multiple laboratory studies have found a delay in fracture healing in diabetic animal models [38–41]. These studies further noted that uncontrolled diabetes resulted in a much greater delay in healing compared with insulin-treated animals [38]. Physiologically, the delay in fracture healing may be related to a decrease in type I, type II, and type X collagen synthesis in the fracture callus [42–44]. Furthermore, laboratory studies have found that treatment with insulin and adequate glucose control corrects the alterations in collagen metabolism [42]. The combination of metabolic alterations, neuropathy, and angiopathy predisposes diabetic patients to delayed fracture healing.

Neurovascular changes and autonomic dysfunction may result secondarily in altered osteoclastic activity and bone turnover [45,46]. Hyperemia secondary to peripheral neuropathy results in increased osteoclastic bone resorption without an increase in osteoblastic activity. Studies have found that the bisphosphonates (pamidronate and alendronate) may improve bone mineral density in diabetic patients [47,48]. The osteopenia predisposes the patient to fracture subluxations, delayed fracture healing, and mechanical failure of hardware in surgically treated patients. If osteopenic bone results in a loss of fracture fixation, revision to a more stable construct may be necessary. Additionally, these patients should be protected from weight-bearing stresses for prolonged periods.

Delayed wound healing

Wound healing is a major concern when contemplating open reduction and internal fixation (ORIF) of an ankle fracture in a diabetic patient.

Wound complications can be a source of serious limb-threatening morbidity and even mortality in the diabetic. The hyperglycemia intrinsic to diabetes and the angiopathic complications of diabetes results in a reduction in wound healing potential.

Hyperglycemia results in the nonenzymatic glycosylation of proteins throughout the body. Glycosylation of structural proteins such as collagens, enzymes, surface integrins, and receptors alters the mechanics of wound healing. The inflammatory process, which produces critical growth factors and promotes cellular recruitment and maturity, can be affected greatly by these structural alterations. The combination of tissue hypoxia resulting from the small- and large-vessel angiopathy, increased viscosity of hyperglycemic blood, impaired oxygen delivery by the glycosylated hemoglobin, and fibroblastic dysfunction (decreased migration, replication, and collagen synthesis) creates an unfavorable local environment for healing [44,49,50]. Furthermore, systemic host factors such as smoking, hyperlipidemia, obesity, malnutrition and unrecognized neuropathy with delays in treatment result in a severely compromised environment for wound healing [37,51].

In addition to limitations in operative wound healing, neuropathic ulcers can take long periods to heal and may become infected and jeopardize the prognosis of the affected limb. A preoperative assessment to optimize blood glucose levels, improve nutrition, and assess angiopathy accurately may help limit wound healing complications. Despite meticulous examination and preoperative planning, wound complications may still develop. Wound complications must be recognized and treated expeditiously, with the ultimate goal being avoidance of osteomyelitis and the even more feared below-knee amputation. These wounds should be treated aggressively with debridement, vacuum-assisted closure, or flap coverage.

Immune dysfunction

Flynn and colleagues [52] noted that the diabetic patient with an ankle fracture had an increased risk of infection over the nondiabetic patient with an ankle fracture. The infection rate in the nondiabetic patients was 8% (6 of 73) compared with 32% (8 of 25) in diabetic patients. This result was similar to that reported by Low and Tan [53]. The hyperglycemic and hypoxic environment of the diabetic wound contributes to an increased susceptibility to infection. This occurs via a reduced immune cell ability to attach and migrate into diabetic wounds and a reduction in the release of protective enzymes and oxidative defense mechanisms. Subsequently, bacterial enzymes and metalloproteinases degrade wound healing proteins such as fibrin and various growth factors [44]. The chemotactic and phagocytic function of granulocytes and macrophages is impaired in diabetics with poorly controlled disease, thus decreasing the ability to clear necrotic debris and release critical anabolic growth factor [54].

Nonoperative treatment versus operative treatment

Diabetic patients who sustain an ankle fracture are at increased risk of complications with or without operative intervention. Kristiansen [55,56] reported on two series of ankle fractures showing more postoperative wound infections, Charcot neuroarthropathy, and delayed healing in diabetic patients compared with nondiabetic patients. Several other findings have substantiated this [52,57,58]. Alternatively, nonoperative treatment of ankle fractures in diabetics does not eliminate complications. This finding may be because of selection bias, because the highest-risk patients with the greatest number of comorbidities often are selected for nonoperative treatment. It is agreed generally that displaced ankle fractures should be treated with operative intervention, striving to achieve an anatomic reduction with skeletal stability. Nondisplaced ankle fractures potentially may be treated nonoperatively; however, Connolly and Csencsitz reported unsatisfactory results in 67% (four of six) of patients treated with a nonoperative protocol [57]. Of these patients, one required amputation for uncontrolled sepsis, another had severe neuropathic arthropathy requiring long-term bracing, and two patients with early weight bearing underwent fusions to treat neuropathic arthropathy. A fifth patient sustained bilateral minimally displaced bimalleolar ankle fractures with one side treated nonoperatively and the other subsequent injury treated operatively. The ankle with closed reduction and casting progressed rapidly to Charcot neuroarthropathy, whereas the operatively fixed ankle had a good result. McCormack and Leith [59] noted that five of seven diabetic patients treated nonoperatively for their ankle fractures resulted in malunions. They did not find a significant difference between insulin-dependent diabetics and non–insulin-dependent diabetics in overall complications. Furthermore, they stated that these malunions caused few symptoms and that all patients had functional lower limbs. Interestingly, in a rebuttal letter by Connolly [60], it was suggested that the malunions of McCormack and Leith in fact may have been Charcot neuroarthropathy.

Blotter and coworkers [58] noted a three-fold increase in postoperative complications in diabetic patients and stressed the role of patient education and postoperative compliance in improvement of outcomes. Flynn and colleagues [52] observed that patients with the greatest surgical risk (swelling, ecchymosis, neuropathy, poorly compliant, peripheral vascular disease [PVD]) were also the most difficult to treat in a cast because of skin complications. Their solution to this dilemma includes a multidisciplinary team approach to provide strict glucose control, patient education, identification of comorbidities, proper total-contact casting techniques, and frequent follow-up evaluations.

Lillmars and Meister [61] performed a meta-analysis of five series of ankle fractures in diabetics, which found 356 ankle fractures, of which, 127 diabetic patients were treated with ORIF. The overall complication rate in diabetic patients treated by ORIF was 29% with an overall infection rate of 25%. In the diabetics treated by nonoperative protocols, the complication rate was 83% with an infection rate of 40%. In nondiabetic controls the overall infection rate was only 6%. It was noted that infections developed more frequently in diabetics treated operatively and were more severe than in the nondiabetic controls. The overall amputation rate in diabetics with ankle fractures was 5% compared with 0.4% in nondiabetics. Diabetic patients with PVD and neuropathy were at increased risk for complications regardless of method of treatment.

Jones and coauthors [62] attempted to determine which factors were related to increased risk of complications in diabetic patients with rotational ankle fractures. They reviewed retrospectively 42 diabetic patients matched to 42 control patients with at least a 6 month follow-up [62]. They noted that diabetic patients without known comorbidities (neuropathy, nephropathy, PVD) at the time of fracture did not have an increased rate of complications compared with nondiabetics with ankle fractures. However, patients with one or more diabetic comorbidities (especially a history of Charcot neuroarthropathy in a different joint) had more complications and were more likely to have long-term needs for bracing. Infection developed in 19% of these patients, and 33% had complications of fracture healing (malunion, nonunion, or Charcot). Patients with diabetes for a longer duration, history of Charcot, or insulin dependency had a worse prognosis after ankle fracture. A history of Charcot neuroarthropathy was the only significant risk factor for perioperative infection. Complications of fracture healing were statistically more frequent in patients with a history of Charcot, a longer duration of diabetes, use of insulin, presence of nephropathy, or presence of sensory neuropathy. The same comorbidities, including retinopathy, correlated with a need for continued bracing at 6 months after fracture. They noted that patient age, patient gender, type of fracture, and method of treatment (operative versus nonoperative) did not correlate with any particular complication or overall complication rate.

Management of ankle fractures in diabetics

History

Management of the diabetic with an ankle fracture begins with a thorough history. The mechanism of injury and timing of injury are very important, although some patients may not have a known injury to the ankle. Determination of the energy of the mechanism (high or low) will help with expected soft tissue complications and swelling. Likewise, it will help with an understanding of the bone quality (osteopenic or porotic), because a low energy mechanism linked to a complex fracture may indicate poor bone quality. Also, if a patient fractured an ankle more than 24 hours before presentation and has continued to ambulate on that fracture, neuropathy can be inferred. A history of Charcot arthropathy, neuropathy, nephropathy, retinopathy, insulin use, previous foot ulcers, peripheral vascular disease, smoking, weight gain, elevated HbA_{1c}, or noncompliance with medical care should be explored.

Physical

The physical examination should begin with inspection of the integrity and quality of the soft tissue envelope. Lacerations and tension on the skin indicative of a pending or already open fracture need to be addressed urgently. Fractures tenting the skin need to be reduced and re-examined for evidence of tissue pressure necrosis. Tense swelling with loss of skin creases or fracture blisters may indicate compartment syndrome or a need to delay operative fixation to avoid wound complications.

The presence or absence of pedal pulses should be documented. If pulses are nonpalpable or asymmetric, noninvasive vascular assessment such as Dopplers and ABIs should be performed. The latter may be difficult in the acute setting because of pain and swelling, and abnormalities noted on noninvasive examination can be evaluated further by T_cPo_2 measurements if available. Transcutaneous oximetry is particularly useful because it also assesses the microcirculation and can be measured directly at the site of the planned incision. If T_cPo_2 is less than 30 mm Hg, vascular consultation should be obtained preoperatively. Evaluation for revascularization procedures should be considered before operative intervention and may be done concomitant with operative fracture fixation.

Protective sensation should be evaluated using a 5.07/10 g Semmes-Weinstein monofilament under the great toe, third toe, and fifth toe. Further neurologic examination should assess motor function and reflexes. Intrinsic atrophy may present as claw toes. Neuropathic autonomic dysfunction may present as loss of skin integrity with dry cracking skin.

Planning

As mentioned above, prompt reduction and splinting should be done for displaced fractures to relieve any tension on overlying skin. The splint should be well padded and the foot elevated to limit swelling. Preoperative and perioperative medical care should be done via a multidisciplinary team approach. Preoperative assessment of blood glucose control; metabolic dysfunction; and electrolyte imbalances, heart disease, hypertension, peripheral vascular disease, and nephropathy is critical to the care of the diabetic patient undergoing surgery. Careful control of blood glucose, especially in times of stress such as perioperatively, may require continuous insulin infusions even in non–insulin-dependent patients.

Fracture management

The goals of treatment for an ankle fracture, whether operative or nonoperative, are to achieve a congruent and stable joint, restore function, and prevent complications that could lead to limb loss or death. Except in extenuating circumstances, surgical fixation of unstable ankle fracture is the treatment of choice. The principles that have been associated with a successful outcome include more rigid fixation to withstand stresses that the insensate diabetic may unknowingly apply, prolonged non–weight-bearing status, and more vigilant follow-up. A good rule is to double the amount of fixation, double the time of non–weight bearing, and double the usual number of office visits. If a nonoperative approach is undertaken for a stable, nondisplaced isolated lateral or medial malleolus fracture, non–weight bearing in a total contact cast for 3 months is advisable. Weekly or biweekly radiographs are necessary to monitor the stability of the fracture (Figs. 1 and 2). Any subtle evidence of subluxation should be treated with operative management if the soft tissues permit open surgery. Protected weight bearing in a total contact cast or brace is recommended for an additional 2 to 3 months after fracture union. Further use of protective braces may be necessary after this.

In nonosteopenic diabetic patients without peripheral neuropathy, standard small fragment fixation with a lag screw and plate fixation of the fibula and cancellous screws for the medial malleolus may be used. These patients still should have a prolonged period of non–weight bearing. In patients with severe osteopenia or neuropathy, more rigid fixation should be used. Perry and coworkers [63] recommend a 4.5-mm dynamic compression plate (DCP)

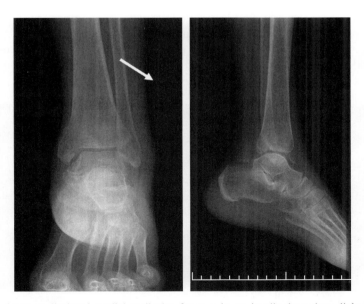

Fig. 1. Acute undisplaced medial malleolus fracture in an insulin-dependent diabetic with peripheral neuropathy. Initial treatment included immobilization in a Jones dressing with a U splint and posterior splint.

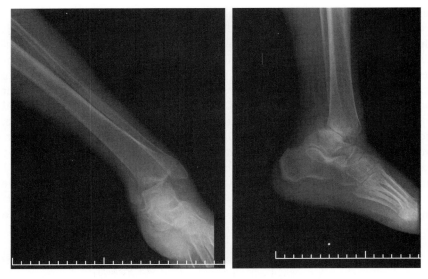

Fig. 2. Follow-up x-ray 8 days later shows displacement and subluxation despite immobilization in the U and posterior splints. The soft tissue envelope was compromised because of the instability and subluxation.

for lateral fixation with syndesmotic screw fixation. Schon and Marks [64] further support the use of multiple syndesmotic screws in patients with neuropathy and a displaced ankle fracture (Figs. 3 and 4). The risk with these larger, more rigid fixation techniques is that bulky hardware may necessitate removal if prominent or if wound dehiscence occurs. Also, if medial

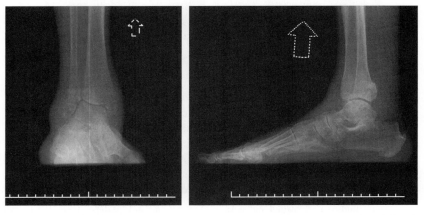

Fig. 3. Seven-week-old fracture treated nonoperatively shows nonunion and valgus deformity. This patient has diabetic neuropathy.

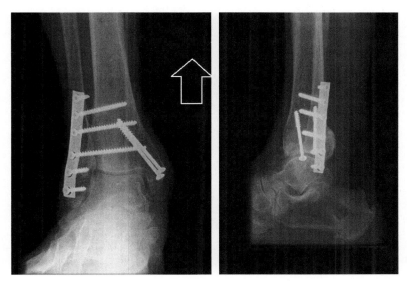

Fig. 4. Nine-month follow-up x-ray after ORIF using multiple syndesmotic screws. No collapse of the ankle joint has occurred, and the fracture has healed.

cancellous screw fixation does not achieve stable fixation, these screws can be advanced obliquely into the tibial far cortex. A tension band wiring or plating technique may be used to enhance medial fixation.

For very unstable fractures or fracture dislocations, further external and internal fixation strategies may be used. Jani and colleagues [65] described the use of transarticular fixation of the subtalar and tibiotalar joints alone or in combination with traditional Association for the Study of Internal Fixation (AO) techniques of internal fixation. If an Achilles tendon contracture is present, a percutaneous triple step tendon lengthening can be considered . Smooth 1/8- or 5/32-in axial Steinmann pins are placed retrograde through the plantar surface of the calcaneus and engaging the distal tibial cortex to prevent proximal migration. The pins are cut short beneath the skin, and a tamp is used to drive the pins far enough to avoid prominence on the plantar surface and subsequent ulceration. The pins then are removed at approximately 3 to 4 months (Figs. 5 and 6).

External fixators may be used to provide additional stability without the use of bulky internal hardware. An external fixator also removes the need for casting or splinting and allows for close inspection of skin and wounds. Various forms of external fixation are available to include half-pin configurations (ie, Delta or unilateral frames) versus small-wire circular fixation, which stabilize the ankle in multiple planes. External fixators can remain in place until the fracture heals. Unilateral frames with half-pin constructs typically have a higher pin tract infection rate than small-wire circular frames and do not provide the same level of stability as afforded by circular

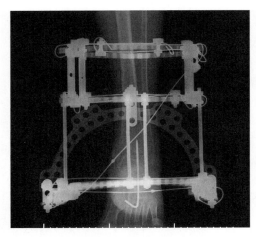

Fig. 5. The use of circular small wire external fixation with an intramedullary Steinman pin. This is the same patient shown in Figs. 1 and 2. Because of the soft tissue compromise, the medial fragment was stabilized with a percutaneously placed olive wire restoring the anatomy.

frames. Supplementary external fixation can remain in place for 6 to 12 weeks if skin conditions permit.

Once the external fixator is removed, total contact casting is recommended. Protected weight bearing is permitted only after radiographic evidence of fracture healing (usually at 12 weeks). This may be in another total contact cast or a removable boot in compliant patients. External fixation may also increase the patient's compliance with a non–weight-bearing protocol.

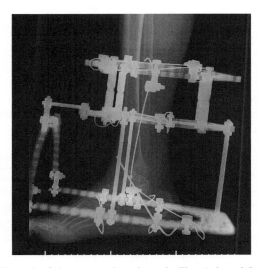

Fig. 6. Lateral radiograph of the same patient shown in Figs. 1, 2, and 5. The intramedullary pin is seen with reduction of the joint.

Compliance with a non–weight-bearing protocol can also be achieved without external fixation by placement of a long leg cast in 30° of knee flexion.

Summary

Treatment of the diabetic patient with an ankle fracture presents a unique set of challenges to the surgeon. The care of these patients should follow a multidisciplinary approach with a team of orthopedic and vascular surgeons, internists, anesthesiologists, nurses, and diabetic educators. Meticulous preoperative planning, intraoperative technique, and postoperative care can decrease potential limb-threatening complications; however, complications will occur despite excellent care. Early recognition and treatment of perioperative complications is imperative. These patients require close attention for long periods, and the surgeon should plan on building a strong relationship with these patients.

References

[1] Centers for Disease Control Website statistics. Available at: http://www.cdc.gov/diabetes/statistics/prev/. Accessed 2003.

[2] Mayfield J. Diagnosis and classification of diabetes mellitus: new criteria. Am Fam Physician 1998;58(6):1355–62, 1369–70.

[3] Bauer M, Bergstrom B, Hemborg A, et al. Malleolar fractures: nonoperative versus operative treatment. A controlled study. Clin Orthop Relat Res 1985;Oct(199):17–27.

[4] Koval KJ, Lurie J, Zhou W, et al. Ankle fractures in the elderly: what you get depends on where you live and who you see. J Orthop Trauma 2005;19(9):635–9.

[5] Ganesh SP, Pietrobon R, Cecilio WA, et al. The impact of diabetes on patient outcomes after ankle fracture. J Bone Joint Surg Am 2005;87(8):1712–8.

[6] Cofield RH, Morrison MJ, Beabout JW. Diabetic neuroarthropathy in the foot: patient characteristics and patterns of radiographic change. Foot Ankle 1983;4(1):15–22.

[7] Kumar S, Ashe HA, Parnell LN, et al. The prevalence of foot ulceration and its correlates in type 2 diabetic patients: a population-based study. Diabet Med 1994;11(5):480–4.

[8] Singh N, Armstrong DG, Lipsky BA. Preventing foot ulcers in patients with diabetes. JAMA 2005;293(2):217–28.

[9] Wunderlich RP, Peters EJ, Bosma J, et al. Pathophysiology and treatment of painful diabetic neuropathy of the lower extremity. South Med J 1998;91(10):894–8.

[10] Armstrong DG. Loss of protective sensation: a practical evidence-based definition. J Foot Ankle Surg 1999;38:79–80.

[11] Reiber GE, Vileikyte L, Boyko EJ, et al. Causal pathways for incident lower-extremity ulcers in patients with diabetes from two settings. Diabetes Care 1999;22:157–62.

[12] Young MJ, Breddy JL, Veves A, et al. The prediction of diabetic neuropathic foot ulceration using vibration perception thresholds: a prospective study. Diabetes Care 1994;17:557–60.

[13] Armstrong DG. The 10-g monofilament: the diagnostic divining rod for the diabetic foot? Diabetes Care 2000;23:887.

[14] Boyko EJ, Ahroni JH, Stensel V, et al. A prospective study of risk factors for diabetic foot ulcer: the Seattle Diabetic Foot Study. Diabetes Care 1999;22:1036–42.

[15] Rith-Najarian SJ, Stolusky T, Gohdes DM. Identifying diabetic patients at risk for lower extremity amputation in a primary health care setting. Diabetes Care 1992;15:1386–9.

[16] Pham H, Armstrong DG, Harvey C, et al. Screening techniques to identify the at risk patients for developing diabetic foot ulcers in a prospective multicenter trial. Diabetes Care 2000;23: 606–11.

[17] Smieja M, Hunt DL, Edelman D, et al. International Cooperative Group for Clinical Examination Research. Clinical examination for the detection of protective sensation in the feet of diabetic patients. J Gen Intern Med 1999;14:418–24.

[18] Armstrong DG, Lavery LA, Vela SA, et al. Choosing a practical screening instrument to identify patients at risk for diabetic foot ulceration. Arch Intern Med 1998;158:289–92.

[19] Perkins BA, Olaleye D, Zinman B, et al. Simple screening tests for peripheral neuropathy in the diabetes clinic. Diabetes Care 2001;24:250–6.

[20] Bibbo C, Lin SS, Beam HA, et al. Complications of ankle fractures in diabetic patients. Orthop Clin North Am 2001;32(1):113–33.

[21] Edmonds ME. The diabetic foot: pathophysiology and treatment. Clin Endocrinol Metab 1986;15(4):889–916.

[22] Slowman-Kovacs SD, Braunstein EM, Brandt KD. Rapidly progressive Charcot arthropathy following minor joint trauma in patients with diabetic neuropathy. Arthritis Rheum 1990;33(3):412–7.

[23] Finsterbush A, Friedman B. The effect of sensory denervation on rabbits' knee joints. A light and electron microscopic study. J Bone Joint Surg Am 1975;57(7):949–56.

[24] Holmes GB Jr, Hill N. Fractures and dislocations of the foot and ankle in diabetics associated with Charcot joint changes. Foot Ankle Int 1994;15(4):182–5.

[25] Novo S. Classification, epidemiology, risk factors, and natural history of peripheral arterial disease. Diabetes Obes Metab 2002;4(Suppl 2):S1–6.

[26] Costigan WB, Thordarson DB. Surgical management of ankle fractures in diabetics. Monterey (CA): American Orthopaedic Foot and Ankle Society; 1997.

[27] American Diabetes Association. Peripheral arterial disease in people with diabetes. Diabetes Care 2003;26:3333–41.

[28] Lobmann R, Ambrosch A, Schultz G, et al. Expression of matrix-metalloproteinases and their inhibitors in the wounds of diabetic and non-diabetic patients. Diabetologia 2002;45: 1011–6.

[29] Geerlings SE, Hoepelman AI. Immune dysfunction in patients with diabetes mellitus (DM). FEMS Immunol Med Microbiol 1999;26:259–65.

[30] Joshi N, Caputo GM, Weitekamp MR, et al. Infections in patients with diabetes mellitus. N Engl J Med 1999;341:1906–12.

[31] Ballard JL, Eke CC, Bunt TJ, et al. A prospective evaluation of transcutaneous oxygen measurements in the management of diabetic foot problems. J Vasc Surg 1995;22(4):485–90.

[32] Bunt TJ, Holloway GA. TcPO2 as an accurate predictor of therapy in limb salvage. Ann Vasc Surg 1996;10(3):224–7.

[33] Bongard O, Krahenbuhl B. Predicting amputation in severe ischaemia. The value of transcutaneous PO2 measurement. J Bone Joint Surg Br 1988;70(3):465–7.

[34] Sumpio BE, Lee T, Blume PA. Vascular evaluation and arterial reconstruction of the diabetic foot. Clin Podiatr Med Surg 2003;20:689–708.

[35] Faglia E, Mantero M, Caminiti M, et al. Extensive use of peripheral angioplasty, particularly infrapopliteal, in the treatment of ischaemic diabetic foot ulcers: clinical results of a multicentric study of 221 consecutive diabetic subjects. J Intern Med 2002;252:225–32.

[36] Loder RT. The influence of diabetes mellitus on the healing of closed fractures. Clin Orthop 1988;July(232):210–6.

[37] Sinacore DR. Acute Charcot arthropathy in patients with diabetes mellitus: healing times by foot location. J Diabetes Complications 1998;12(5):287–93.

[38] Dixit PK, Ekstrom RA. Retardation of bone fracture healing in experimental diabetes. Indian J Med Res 1987;85:426–35.

[39] Harris BH, Powers J, Shaftan GW, et al. Vascular component of fracture healing in experimental diabetes. Surg Forum 1968;19:450–1.

[40] Herbsman H, Kwon K, Shaftan GW, et al. The influence of systemic factors on fracture healing. J Trauma 1966;6(1):75–85.
[41] Herbsman H, Powers JC, Hirschman A, et al. Retardation of fracture healing in experimental diabetes. J Surg Res 1968;8(9):424–31.
[42] Umpierrez GE, Zlatev T, Spanheimer RG. Correction of altered collagen metabolism in diabetic animals with insulin therapy. Matrix 1989;9(4):336–42.
[43] Spanheimer RG, Umpierrez GE, Stumpf V. Decreased collagen production in diabetic rats. Diabetes 1988;37(4):371–6.
[44] Stadelmann WK, Digenis AG, Tobin GR. Impediments to wound healing. Am J Surg 1998 Aug; 176(2A Suppl):39S–47S.
[45] Edmonds ME, Clarke MB, Newton S, et al. Increased uptake of bone radiopharmaceutical in diabetic neuropathy. Q J Med 1985;57(224):843–55.
[46] Gough A, Abraha H, Li F, et al. Measurement of markers of osteoclast and osteoblast activity in patients with acute and chronic diabetic Charcot neuroarthropathy. Diabet Med 1997;14(7):527–31.
[47] Jude EB, Selby PL, Burgess J, et al. Bisphosphonates in the treatment of Charcot neuroarthropathy: a double-blind randomised controlled trial. Diabetologia 2001;44(11):2032–7.
[48] Keegan TH, Schwartz AV, Bauer DC, et al, the fracture intervention trial. Effect of alendronate on bone mineral density and biochemical markers of bone turnover in type 2 diabetic women: the fracture intervention trial. Diabetes Care 2004;27(7):1547–53.
[49] Harrelson JM. The diabetic foot: Charcot arthropathy. Instr Course Lect 1996;42:141–6.
[50] Ramasastry SS. Chronic wound problems. Clin Plast Surg 1998;25:367–96.
[51] Mancini L, Ruotolo V. Infection of the diabetic foot. Rays 1997;22(4):544–9.
[52] Flynn JM, Rodriguez-del Rio F, Piza PA. Closed ankle fractures in the diabetic patient. Foot Ankle Int 2000;21(4):311–9.
[53] Low CK, Tan SK. Infection in diabetic patients with ankle fractures. Ann Acad Med Singapore 1995;24(3):353–5.
[54] Nolan CM, Beaty HN, Bagdade JD. Further characterization of the impaired bactericidal function of granulocytes in patients with poorly controlled diabetes. Diabetes 1978;27(9):889–94.
[55] Kristiansen B. Ankle and foot fractures in diabetics provoking neuropathic joint changes. Acta Orthop Scand 1980;51(6):975–9.
[56] Kristiansen B. Results of surgical treatment of malleolar fractures in patients with diabetes mellitus. Dan Med Bull 1983;30(4):272–4.
[57] Connolly JF, Csencsitz TA. Limb threatening neuropathic complications from ankle fractures in patients with diabetes. Clin Orthop 1998;Mar(348):212–9.
[58] Blotter RH, Connolly E, Wasan A, et al. Acute complications in the operative treatment of isolated ankle fractures in patients with diabetes mellitus. Foot Ankle Int 1999;20(11):687–94.
[59] McCormack RG, Leith JM. Ankle fractures in diabetics. Complications of surgical management. J Bone Joint Surg Br 1998;80(4):689–92.
[60] Connolly JF. Ankle fractures in diabetics. J Bone Joint Surg Br 1999;81(2):370.
[61] Lillmars SA, Meister BR. Acute trauma to the diabetic foot and ankle. Curr Opin Orthop 2001;12:100–5.
[62] Jones KB, Maiers-Yelden KA, Marsh JL, et al. Ankle fractures in patients with diabetes mellitus. J Bone Joint Surg Br 2005;87(4):489–95.
[63] Perry MD, Taranow WS, Manoli A 2nd, et al. Salvage of failed neuropathic ankle fractures: use of large-fragment fibular plating and multiple syndesmotic screws. J Surg Orthop Adv 2005;14(2):85–91.
[64] Schon LC, Marks RM. The management of neuroarthropathic fracture-dislocations in the diabetic patient. Orthop Clin North Am 1995;26(2):375–92.
[65] Jani MM, Ricci WM, Borrelli J Jr, et al. A protocol for treatment of unstable ankle fractures using transarticular fixation in patients with diabetes mellitus and loss of protective sensibility. Foot Ankle Int 2003;24(11):838–44.

ELSEVIER
SAUNDERS

Foot Ankle Clin N Am
11 (2006) 865–869

FOOT AND
ANKLE CLINICS

Index

Note: Page numbers of article titles are in **boldface** type.